Your *Natural* PREGNANCY

D0890472

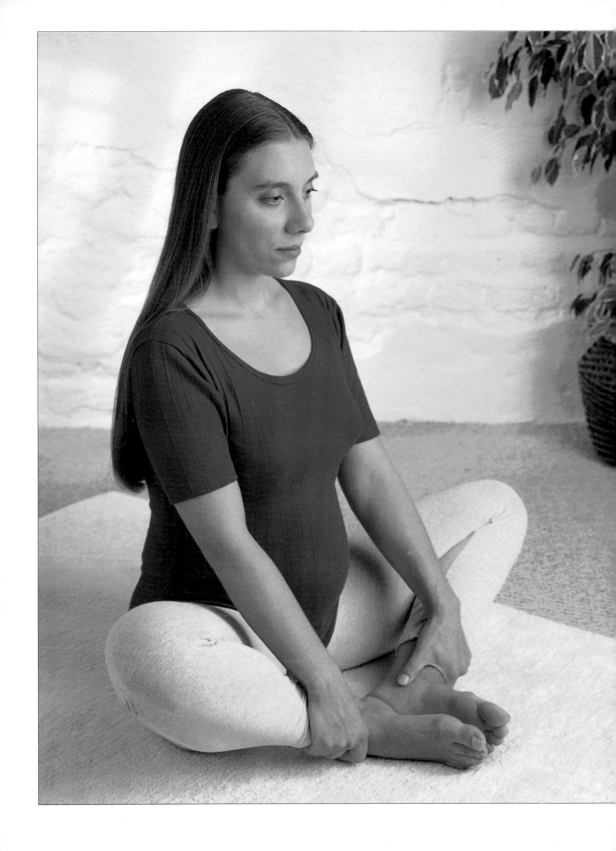

Your *Natural* PREGNANCY
A Guide to Complementary Therapies

ANNE CHARLISH

Consultant: Adriane Fugh-Berman MD

Complementary therapy consultant:
Debbie Shapiro

Photography by Gill Orsman

Ulysses Press

To TH whose qualities and sensitivity as a father
and a man would enrich any woman's life.

Text copyright © Anne Charlish 1995
Photographs copyright © Gill Orsman 1995
Illustrations copyright © Julie Carpenter 1995
This edition copyright © Eddison Sadd Editions 1996

The right of Anne Charlish to be identified as the author of the work has been asserted by
her in accordance with the Copyright, Designs and Patents Act 1988.

Published by: Ulysses Press
P.O. Box 3440
Berkeley, CA 94703–3440

Library of Congress Catalog Card Number: 95-83567

ISBN: 1-56975-059-9

1 3 5 7 9 8 6 4 2

AN EDDISON·SADD EDITION
Edited, designed and produced by
Eddison Sadd Editions Limited
St Chad's House
148 King's Cross Road
London WC1X 9DH

Phototypeset in Baskerville No. 2 and Americana Bold using QuarkXpress
on Apple Macintosh.
Origination by Chroma Graphics Pte Ltd, Singapore.
Printed and bound by BPC Paulton Books Ltd, UK.

Contents

❧

Foreword

The last forty years have seen great improvements in care during pregnancy, resulting in a better outcome for both mother and baby. Certainly the creation of professional bodies to oversee the education and practice of doctors and midwives were important events. And the development of the technology which allows us to see inside the womb with ultrasound has also been remarkable. The secret life of the unborn child, hitherto a mystery, has been explored, and the treatment of the baby in the womb has become a reality.

These developments have been associated with more universal hospital birth, other medical advances and much technological innovation. However, most pregnancies are normal and such degrees of medicalization are now seen as inappropriate from this comfortable standpoint of a more assured, though never guaranteed, good result. Given appropriate professional advice, the mother should be given more choice concerning the events of her pregnancy. This view has been highlighted in a recent UK government report entitled *Changing Childbirth*, which places the woman at the center of care. This dictates a more holistic approach to pregnancy and childbirth which should encompass any technique, customary or complementary.

The move away from the word "alternative" is critical and central to the theme of this book. Many medical professionals and patients alike have become disillusioned with the lack of results achieved by conventional medicine and have seen interesting results from techniques used in different cultures and environments. Of course these techniques or therapies should be honest, with some mechanism to ensure protection of the public from unscrupulous practitioners wishing to exploit the vulnerable. This book offers explanations of how honest therapists practice, thus providing the information necessary to make a more informed choice. In this book, Anne Charlish succeeds in providing a comprehensive source of information about complementary techniques. She considers, systematically, the methods and their applications, including information on remedies and exercises you can adopt safely. There is a sense of balance about the relationship between these methods and more mainstream medical care. The approach she has taken is pragmatic and realistic.

Although not subjected to scientific scrutiny, the role of complementary therapies alongside conventional methods is promoted by more and more doctors. Homeopathy and acupuncture have been used effectively in pregnancy and labor, and relaxation techniques akin to massage, meditation and yoga have found a place in prenatal preparation classes. The obvious conclusion that physical well-being and psychological well-being are inextricably linked has become an accepted medical principle. These techniques and therapies help the pregnant mother to attain the best possible health so that she is better equipped to deal with labor and with her newborn baby.

This book is very timely given the principles of *Changing Childbirth*, and will play a role in providing mothers with the information necessary to make clear choices. Choice of a specific therapy can be made to suit the needs of the mother in terms of complaint and lifestyle, and the focus of health care can return to how people can help themselves. This book will be helpful to professionals and couples alike, and the inclusion of addresses for the relevant organizations is particularly useful.

Donald Gibb, Consultant Obstetrician,
King's College Hospital, London, England, 1994

Introduction

The intention of this book is to bring together, within a sound medical framework, the many benefits that the complementary therapies can offer the pregnant woman and her partner. Some of these benefits are substantial. For example, herbal teas and tinctures are useful in helping prepare for an easier birth; and aromatherapy massage can relieve pain, cramps and stretch marks; an osteopathy treatment can quickly banish the chronic and characteristic backache of pregnancy; naturopathy will treat breast problems, constipation, heartburn and a host of other difficulties, while homeopathy will help balance your entire system making pregnancy far more enjoyable.

In *Your Natural Pregnancy*, I have sought to provide you with information to help you through conventional prenatal classes and conventional hospital delivery or a home birth. The complementary therapies outlined here can be used as an important and integral part of your pregnancy without you having to cut yourself off from the best that medical knowledge has to offer.

Once you have this knowledge and you are in a position to appreciate the reasons for and the possible outcomes of prenatal and hospital delivery routines, you are in the best possible situation to make informed choices. Never shrink from discussing problems that arise during your pregnancy both with the complementary therapists of your choice and your obstetrician, family practitioner or midwife.

The tremendous resistance shown by allopathic (conventional) doctors to complementary therapies is at last beginning to break down. In the United States, some doctors themselves practice acupuncture, homeopathy, herbalism or hypnosis. Some do, however, still view these therapies as ineffective and potentially dangerous; you need to be fully aware of this view in order to obtain the best possible care. Do not hesitate to discuss your wishes and views with the various people responsible for your care. Should you discover that they are unsympathetic to your views, do not simply turn away, perhaps skipping prenatal checks altogether; discuss the matter. You may decide between you that there is another midwife or consultant within the same hospital who would be more responsive to your views or needs and thus better placed to look after you.

One of the most frequent complaints made by pregnant women is that there is not enough time allowed to ask questions or discuss things. In this case, ask the person you wish to speak to for a special appointment outside of their clinic sessions.

Conventional health care professionals and complementary health therapists alike can provide a tremendous contribution to making your pregnancy and delivery healthy, happy and safe. It is up to you to seek out the benefits. The complementary therapists are more likely to be able to give you the time and emotional support that you may wish for; this is partly because you are paying for their time. The acupuncturist or the homeopath, for example, is not beset with too-long lists of patients all to be seen that afternoon. These therapists set their own pace, often allowing up to an hour for each consultation.

Your Natural Pregnancy contains all those therapies which I believe can offer substantial and worthwhile benefits to the pregnant woman (or to the woman hoping to be so). Part One outlines each therapy, describing the theory and principles and sets it within the context of pregnancy. Part Two takes you through the stages of conception, the three trimesters of pregnancy, the birth and the period immediately following the delivery of your baby. There are also a number of charts throughout the book which will allow you to choose at a glance the therapies which may be useful and enjoyable for you at each stage of pregnancy. In addition, there is a quick reference chart on pages 153–56 which will enable you to see which of the complementary therapies can deal with a particular ailment or condition. You will see that most of the common complaints of pregnancy can be treated with a number of therapies.

If this is your first pregnancy, I hope that this book fulfils its intentions in achieving for you an informed, stress-free pregnancy and delivery through the judicious use of whatever combination of complementary therapies appeals to you: do remember that the therapies can not only complement your orthodox care but they can also complement each other. So pick out those that appeal to you and your partner and those that may be able to resolve any particular problem you may have.

For those women having a second or third child, I hope that this book will give you the kind of information that you wish had been available during your earlier pregnancies and deliveries. The information collected here should improve the quality of your pregnancy and delivery, your feelings and your state of health in particular, and also resolve any specific problems that you experienced during previous pregnancies and deliveries.

I should like to wish you a fulfilling and joyful pregnancy, followed by the birth of a healthy and beautiful child.

Anne Charlish, Sussex, England, 1994

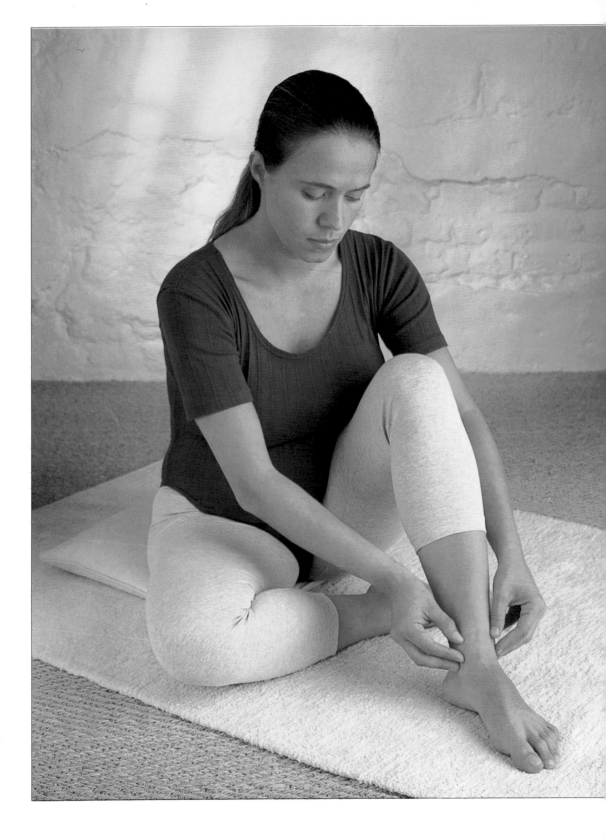

Part One

The Therapies

※

P art One of this book is devoted to describing the complementary therapies as well as providing sections on diet and healthy eating that are most relevant to the woman who is pregnant or who is hoping to be so. The therapies selected are naturopathy, herbalism, homeopathy, massage, aromatherapy, acupuncture, acupressure, shiatsu, reflexology, osteopathy, craniosacral therapy, chiropractic, Alexander technique, yoga, meditation, visualization, hypnotherapy and color therapy.

The theory and principles, together with the historical origins of each therapy are described. Both the role of the therapy in pregnancy, and how it can benefit you, are fully explained. You will discover what to expect in a consultation with each type of therapist, what you may expect to learn and how you may put the therapy into practice at home, either on your own or with your partner. Some of these therapies are deeply luxurious, fun and easy to learn. Start with a sensual aromatherapy treatment, for example. It is important not to exceed the stated dose for any of the treatments and to consult your therapist if you experience any problems. Never ignore any of the danger signs of pregnancy listed on page 85: if you experience any of these symptoms, consult your doctor or the hospital immediately.

Diet

❧

Looking after yourself properly, both before and during pregnancy, is by far the most important thing you can do for the welfare of your baby, and one of the most important aspects of taking good care of yourself is eating well. Not only your health, but your baby's health is entirely dependent on what you eat and drink at this stage. Eating a good diet is obviously important for your own health, whether you are pregnant or not, but during pregnancy it is your health, regardless of other factors such as age, which has the greatest effect on your developing baby.

Before Conceiving

If you are not already pregnant, you might find the following information helpful. Certainly, if you prepare for pregnancy, you will have less reason to worry about your health and that of your baby. It is therefore important to think carefully about your diet before you decide to conceive. An improvement in your daily diet can make a dramatic improvement to your health almost immediately, especially if you have not paid much attention to it before. Ask yourself the following questions to see if there is any room for improvement. Do you skip breakfast or snack throughout the day? Do you eat cookies and chocolate instead of a piece of fresh fruit? Do you eat junk food rather than cooking fresh food? Do you drink a lot of sodas? If you answer "yes" to most of these questions, you may need to rethink your eating habits now. It is vital to strengthen your immune system before conception in order to ward off ailments that could occur during pregnancy; keep in mind that many drugs, even for common ailments, cannot be taken during pregnancy.

Diet and Fertility

Fertility depends on a great many factors, including your age, your general health, timing intercourse with ovulation and your stress levels. Good diet is therefore only one factor, but it is obviously a major one. Diet has a profound effect on fertility; for example, there is evidence to suggest that the number of births declines during times of food shortage.

There are several vitamins and minerals that are known to increase fertility in both women and men. They will not instantly solve all fertility problems, but they will maximize the fertility of both you and your partner. There are degrees of fertility and anything you can do to increase your chances of conception will not only help you get pregnant when you want to, but will also increase your chances of having a trouble-free pregnancy and a healthy baby.

For both men and women, vitamin E is of importance, along with zinc. Vitamin B6 is essential to the fertility of women whereas vitamin C is especially important in male fertility (*see chart Important Vitamins During Pregnancy on page 17 for food sources of these particular vitamins*).

During Pregnancy

To ensure that your pregnancy develops in as healthy a way as possible, it is most important to nourish yourself well. In order to do this, it is not so much a question of following a special diet as of eating a good variety of all the right foods. If you become deficient in any vitamins or minerals, this will affect not only your health but also your ability to support the pregnancy and the health of your baby.

Weight Gain

It may sound obvious, but it is very important: during pregnancy, you *should* gain weight. Your appetite will undoubtedly increase while you are pregnant, which is nature's way of telling you to eat enough. Until quite recently some medical advice suggested that pregnant women should not "eat for two." This led many pregnant women to eat inadequate amounts of food, so afraid were they of gaining weight. Needless to say, this has led to pregnancies fraught with problems, difficult labors and underweight, poorly babies.

Mothers who gain a reasonable amount of weight, on the other hand, tend to have easier pregnancies and labors, with a lower incidence of miscarriage and neo-natal deaths (deaths at around the time of delivery). Heavier babies usually tend to be healthier, and they are also, as a rule, better able to resist common childhood ailments and infections.

A word of warning, however; mothers who gain far too much weight can develop diabetes in pregnancy. It is important to check the urine for sugar during pregnancy.

Why Gain Weight?

A pregnant woman needs to lay down fat early in her pregnancy in preparation for producing milk and breastfeeding. These stores of fat will remain after delivery but will usually vanish gradually with breastfeeding and exercise. But not all the weight gain is made up of fat. The placenta, the fluids surrounding the baby and the baby itself, account for over half your total weight gain.

During pregnancy, the volume of blood manufactured by your body is increased by about 1.5 litres (2.5 pints). This extra blood, which also contributes to your weight gain, is needed by the uterus, the breasts and the other vital organs to sustain and support a healthy pregnancy.

How Much Weight?

Most women gain between 9 and 13.5kg (20–30lb) during pregnancy. Obviously, the amount and rate of weight gain varies from individual to individual, thus making it difficult and wrong to lay down any hard-and-fast rules about how much weight you should or should not put on. It is clear, though, that no pregnant woman should be on a weight-reducing diet, an action which could be harmful to both mother and baby.

The woman who is already overweight before her pregnancy may not need to gain as much weight during pregnancy as the woman who is underweight, but she should certainly not be thinking about slimming.

Weight Gain in Pregnancy

Your total weight gain during pregnancy is made up as follows:

Baby	*38%*
Placenta	*9%*
Amniotic fluid	*11%*
Increased weight of uterus and breasts	*20%*
Increased volume of blood	*22%*

A woman who eats what she needs will usually put on weight according to a predictable pattern (*see Rate of Weight Gain table below*). Your weight will be monitored throughout your pregnancy.

Rate of Weight Gain

However much weight you gain in pregnancy, you will probably gain it at the following rate:

0–12 weeks	*10%*
13–20 weeks	*25%*
21–28 weeks	*45%*
29–36 weeks	*20%*
37–40 weeks	*0%*

Eating Sensibly

It is most important that everything you eat at this time should be good for you and your baby. A healthy diet is not a "quack" diet; quite simply, it should concentrate on fresh, wholesome foods, including fish, lean meat in moderation, and plenty of whole grains, fruit and vegetables. If you have not eaten well before, get into the habit of eating properly now. It will not only give your baby the best possible start in life, it will also instil good habits in you and your partner and eventually your children when they start to select food for themselves.

Listen to your body: if you are eating well, you will feel well. If you are eating badly—junk foods and too many sweet snacks—it will let you know, because the chances are you will frequently feel tired, rundown, sluggish and under the weather. Buy as many organic foods as possible, but if you cannot, at least wash all your fruit and vegetables before you eat them. Some people think that it is a good idea to peel them too, in order to remove as many of the harmful chemicals as possible, but this also removes valuable nutrients. In any case, chemicals that will not wash off will be in the flesh too.

The Vital Nutrients

It is particularly important that you are aware of all the vital nutrients that you need for a healthy, well-balanced diet.

Protein

The recommended daily amount of protein for a non-pregnant woman is 45g. A pregnant woman should increase that amount by about 15g to make a total of 60g daily, the amount necessary for the healthy growth of the fetus and the placenta. Foods that contain about 10g of protein include 225ml (8oz/1 cup) milk, 50g (2oz) chicken, 37g (1.5oz) cheese, 50g (2oz) fish, 37g (1.5oz) lean red meat, 2 eggs, 50g (2oz) nuts, 75g (3oz) tofu and 50g (2oz) legumes.

Carbohydrates

Carbohydrates give you energy. They are found in starchy, bulky foods such as bread, potatoes, rice and pasta, all of which also contain many other important nutrients. Carbohydrates are also found in sugar, which is not recommended in excess, nor are those foods that contain sugar. Cookies and cakes, for example, do little for you or your baby's health and are best avoided, especially if you are putting on too much weight. Try, too, to get used to drinks without added sugar.

It is important to eat whole grains, such as whole grain flour or wholewheat bread and brown rice, rather than white bread and rice. Wholefoods are foods as nature intended them to be and therefore contain the nourishment we need in the most digestible form. Processed and junk foods have had many of the natural nutrients removed and processing does not always replace them.

Carbohydrate-rich foods include whole grain flour bread, root vegetables, particularly potatoes, brown rice, wholewheat pasta cereals, preferably whole oats, hot cereal, muesli and legumes.

Fats

Too much fat should be avoided, whether you are pregnant or not, and your need for fat does not increase during pregnancy. Drink skimmed or semi-skimmed rather than full-fat milk, cut all excess fat off meat, choose fish or poultry rather than red meats, and use less butter or margarine. Try steaming or grilling your foods rather than frying. Over-rich sauces should be avoided too, so keep sauces low in fat by using low-fat yoghurt or fromage frais rather than cream.

It was once thought that polyunsaturated fats (sunflower oil, safflower oil) were best for maintaining cardiovascular health, but the current thinking suggests that mono-unsaturated fats such as olive oil (and olive oil margarine), walnut oil and grapeseed oil are better.

Vitamins

A varied and balanced diet of wholefoods, those in their natural unprocessed state, will ensure a sufficient level of all the vitamins you need without having to resort to supplements. It is much better to get your vitamins from food rather than from supplements. It is impossible to achieve the right balance of vitamins from supplements alone and, in any case, food is the only way to get all the other essential nutrients.

Multivitamin supplements may, however, be advisable before conception and during the first three months of pregnancy. Folic acid and vitamin A are essential to prevent neural tube defects such as spina bifida. If you are worried about the quality of your diet and your vitamin intake, you should talk to your doctor, who may advise you to take certain supplements.

It is important to realize, though, that supplements are just that—extras. No supplement can ever take the place of a healthy well-balanced diet.

Minerals

There are three minerals that are particularly important during pregnancy. These are calcium, iron and zinc.

Calcium is important for the developing fetus's healthy teeth and bone formation which begins between weeks four and six. Calcium is better absorbed during pregnancy than at other times and your baby is unlikely to go short. Although the baby takes what calcium it needs, this may leave you short of it for your own teeth and bones.

Your calcium requirement therefore increases as the baby grows. By week twenty-five, it will have more than doubled in size, so you must eat and drink plenty of calcium-rich foods. Calcium supplements are useful for women who never drink milk, either because they are allergic to it or because they simply do not like it. You can take up to 1200mg of calcium a day, although if you are eating well 600mg should be enough.

Calcium is not absorbed efficiently without vitamin D, which is found in milk, butter and eggs. The body will also manufacture its own vitamin D with exposure to the sun. You can take vitamin D in the form of halibut oil capsules, which also contain vitamin A, but you must take care not to overdo your intake of vitamin A, particularly in pregnancy. Calcium-rich foods include milk, soy milk, yoghurt, leafy green vegetables, nuts, legumes, sesame seeds and sardines.

Iron is required in almost double the quantities when you are pregnant because of the large increase in the volume of blood during pregnancy. It is necessary for the formation of red blood cells which contain a substance called hemoglobin. If you do not have enough hemoglobin in your blood, insufficient oxygen may be carried to your baby which will result in lethargy and tiredness. The baby builds up its own supply of iron in its liver which lasts for several months after the birth. This is very important because milk—the baby's diet for several months—contains virtually no iron.

The body does not absorb iron very easily and needs the assistance of vitamin C (present in fresh fruit and vegetables) which aids absorption. Antacid medicines hinder the absorption of iron, and are therefore best avoided, especially during pregnancy.

Many women are routinely given iron tablets in the second and third trimesters of their pregnancy. This is probably not necessary if you are eating a balanced diet containing many iron-rich foods. One simple way of increasing the iron content of your diet is to use iron cooking pots. If you are at all worried about your iron intake, however, you should talk to your GP (general practitioner) or the medical practitioner you see at your prenatal clinic. Vegetarians and vegans should make sure that their iron levels are monitored. There is also an excellent herbal iron tonic available at health food stores.

Iron-rich foods include red meat, liver, dark molasses, whole grains, legumes, egg yolk, dark green leafy vegetables, raisins, prunes, brewer's yeast and nuts.

Zinc levels often fall dramatically during pregnancy, sometimes by as much as 30 percent. It is essential for fetal bone formation, and an inadequate supply of zinc may lead to a small baby.

Zinc-rich foods include oily fish, wheat germ, brewer's yeast, oysters, meat, walnuts, eggs, pumpkin seeds, molasses, onions, nuts, peas and beans.

Are You Vulnerable?

You may have certain allergies or circumstances which make you more vulnerable during pregnancy. As a result, you may need to be especially careful to eat well when you are pregnant. Some problems you may be concerned with include: allergies to cow's milk, being rundown, being underweight,

Important Vitamins During Pregnancy

Vitamin	Food Source	What It Does
Vitamin A	Oily fish, fish liver oils, milk, margarine, butter, eggs, organ meats, green and yellow vegetables, carrots, eggs, oranges, apricots	Builds up resistance to infection, good for teeth, skin, hair and fingernails, and for the formation of the thyroid gland
Vitamin B1 (thiamine)	Organ meats, brewer's yeast, whole grains, wheat germ, nuts, legumes	Good for digestion, growth, lactation and resistance to illness
Vitamin B2 (riboflavin)	Organ meats, brewer's yeast, whole grains, wheat germ, green vegetables, milk, eggs	Good for eyes and skin and for growth and development of the embryo
Vitamin B3 (niacin)	Organ meats, brewer's yeast, whole grains, wheat germ, green vegetables, fish, eggs, milk, nuts	Builds brain cells and promotes resistance to infection
Vitamin B5 (pantothenic acid)	Organ meats, whole grains, wheat bran, eggs, cheese, nuts	Maintains red blood cells
Vitamin B6 (pyridoxine)	Organ meats, meat, fish, brewer's yeast, whole grains, wheat germ, vegetables, bananas, molasses, eggs, dairy products	Promotes resistance to disease, good for the nerves and promotes the formation of healthy red blood cells
Vitamin B12	Organ meats, red meat, eggs, milk, cheese, fish	Promotes the formation of healthy red blood cells, good for baby's central nervous system
Folic acid (part of B complex, sometimes called Vitamin M)	Green leafy vegetables, lamb's liver, walnuts	Helps cell division, essential for the baby's central nervous system. Deficiency has been linked with brain and spinal cord defects at birth. Women who have previously had a baby with one of these defects are often prescribed folic acid before conception
Vitamin C (ascorbic acid)	Fresh fruits, particularly citrus fruits and strawberries, all fresh vegetables, particularly potatoes, green peppers and tomatoes	Helps resistance to infection, promotes the absorption of iron, builds a strong placenta
Vitamin D (calciferol)	Oily fish, fish liver oils, liver, milk, eggs, butter	Encourages the absorption of calcium, promotes the formation of strong bones
Vitamin E	Most foods, particularly wheat germ, vegetable oils, fish, green leafy vegetables, whole grains and legumes	Promotes the formation of healthy cells
Vitamin K	Green leafy vegetables	Helps maintain good coagulation of blood

suffering a recent miscarriage, smoking or drinking heavily, taking regular medication or having a multiple pregnancy. Let your doctor know about these problems so that you may be referred to a nutritionist if it is considered to be necessary.

Salt

A good, balanced diet should provide plenty of salt, which is present naturally in most foods. Most of us take too much salt in our foods, but pregnant women do not need to reduce their intake of salt.

What to Drink

You should increase your intake of fluids when you are pregnant. This will help with any tendency toward constipation, and will help relieve the strain on your already over-loaded kidneys. Drink plenty of mineral water, but do not drink the carbonated sort if it makes you feel bloated and uncomfortable. Also drink plenty of fresh, unsweetened fruit juices.

Avoid caffeine completely by drinking herbal teas in preference to tea or coffee, or buy decaffeinated tea and coffee. Avoid sweet drinks full of additives and sugar and opt for fruit juices, herb drinks or water in preference to cola and other fizzy drinks that contain chemical colors and flavors. Most authorities agree that it is best to steer clear of alcohol altogether while you are pregnant. If you really want to have an occasional alcoholic drink, stick to wine and dilute it with water.

Foods You Should Avoid

As well as avoiding obvious things like junk food, alcohol, sugars and refined foods, there are several foods which you should avoid during pregnancy, including any foods which may be contaminated with listeria or salmonella, as both of these are dangerous to the baby. Avoid if you can cookies, sweets, cakes, sugar as well as tea and coffee in excess. Also steer clear of highly processed foods containing additives; all unpasteurized cheeses and pâté which can contain listeria. To avoid salmonella do not eat raw or undercooked eggs, foods which contain these and undercooked chicken.

Diet and Morning Sickness

If you suffer from morning sickness in the first three months of pregnancy as many women do, you may find, surprisingly, that food provides relief from nausea. Eat small, frequent snacks and avoid highly spiced food, greasy fried food and rich, creamy dishes. Eating more carbohydrates often seems to help, and you should eat nutritious forms of it, such as whole grain flour bread, rice and potatoes, rather than pastries, cakes and cookies.

Diet and Constipation

There is a tendency to develop constipation in pregnancy. You can help to avoid this by eating plenty of raw fruit and vegetables, whole grains and legumes, all of which are rich in fiber. Drinking plenty of mineral water will also help.

Naturopathy

The cornerstone of naturopathy is the belief that "only nature heals." Many of us practice naturopathy without even realizing it. The person who bathes a sprained wrist in cool water is practicing naturopathy. The person who stops eating to give an upset stomach a rest is practicing naturopathy. And the person with a fever who decides to do nothing more than sweat it out is also practicing it.

In its earliest days, naturopathy was known as the nature cure, which perhaps tells us more about its approach. It consists, quite simply, of encouraging the body to heal itself. The naturopathic way of life means that people take responsibility for their own health. It is a simple approach, based on the following principles, all of them natural, and includes fresh air, sunlight, exercise, rest, good nutrition, hygiene, relaxation and hydrotherapy (water therapy).

Naturopaths believe that the symptoms of disease are no more than indications that toxins have accumulated as a result of leading an unhealthy life. The symptoms show that the body is trying to reject these unhealthy practices. Naturopaths believe, too, that the body has the capability to heal itself, as long as it is properly treated and maintained. Naturopaths, therefore, try to eliminate all obstacles to normal body functioning. These obstacles include poor diet, poor posture and stress.

Largely a preventive regime rather than a treatment for disease, naturopathy takes a simple approach, based to a large extent on common-sense principles. It is a holistic approach, taking into account the whole person: the patient's physical, emotional, biochemical and social condition.

It is thought to be particularly effective against degenerative diseases such as heart disease and arthritis and can greatly help people suffering from various forms of inflammation, such as ulcers, eczema, premenstrual syndrome and rheumatoid arthritis. It can also speed up recovery of flu, the common cold, skin complaints and upset stomachs. And it can have a powerful effect on patients suffering from vague but debilitating conditions—for which there may be no clear medical diagnosis—such as fatigue or anxiety.

Generally speaking, naturopathy works especially well for acute conditions, such as sore throats, colitis, gastritis, bronchitis, piles, digestive and liver problems. But it can also help with chronic and serious conditions, such as tuberculosis. In so far as naturopaths concentrate on the patient rather than the disease, it follows that the success or failure of the therapy depends to a large extent on the patient's ability to heal themselves. A young, vital person will probably react well to treatment for flu or bronchitis, whereas a frail, elderly person suffering from the same complaint may not respond as well.

However, naturopaths do not believe that age is a barrier to naturopathy; patients range from children to old people. There is nothing new about naturopathy. It is an ancient approach, whose origins go back over 2000 years to the Greek physician Hippocrates, who maintained that cures should be as natural as possible and that good health is reliant on eating and exercising sensibly.

Its Role in Pregnancy

During pregnancy, the application of natural principles will boost your body's own healing capabilities and enhance your unborn baby's health and developing immune system. A naturopathic approach is perfectly suited to pregnancy. Good nutrition, which is a cornerstone of naturopathy, is the very foundation of fertility, a good pregnancy and a healthy baby. Naturopaths stress the body's nutritional needs, which are vitally important in pregnancy. It promotes eating foods that are as near as possible to their natural state, retaining a high proportion of their essential nutrients, including vitamins, minerals and enzymes. It promotes eating as many fresh and raw foods as possible, so that these foods are not reduced in quality through cooking and heating. And it discourages the use of additives and junk foods. These are all basic principles at the root of establishing a healthy eating program in pregnancy.

Apart from nutrition, naturopathy also encourages the physical alignment of the body, with good posture, mobile joints and muscles, and a life as devoid of negative stress and tension as possible. All of these principles will help promote a healthy pregnancy and produce a healthy baby.

The Consultation

The therapist will begin the consultation by taking a detailed medical history, in much the same way as orthodox doctors do, but will also ask about the patient's lifestyle, diet and stress factors. The practitioner may want to know how the patient's health is affected by certain changes—such as the weather, the time of day, the time of year—as well as eating and sleeping patterns, menstrual cycle, bowel movements and various things that happen on a day-to-day basis, either at home or at work.

The therapist will then examine the patient, paying particular attention to the patient's heart, lungs, blood pressure and circulation. X-rays may also be taken if they are thought necessary, although if you are pregnant, avoid having any X-rays. A few naturopaths may also use hair analysis and iridology (examination of the irises of the eyes) to provide further information and to help them build up an overall picture of the patient's health.

Hair analysis is useful for determining the levels in the body of some essential minerals, such as selenium, zinc and copper. It is useful, too, for determining the levels of certain toxic minerals, such as lead, aluminium and mercury. Some practitioners will test for these toxic substances, but hair analysis is not an accurate test for any type of allergy.

The naturopath will make a diagnosis taking the whole person into consideration, then will suggest a course of treatment which may include a radical reorganization of the patient's lifestyle. A change in diet is usually the starting point and the naturopath will decide a suitable course of action. This course of action may be described as either *catabolic* or *anabolic*.

Catabolic means, literally, "breaking down." This treatment is best suited to those whose bodies are in a congested or toxic state. A patient who is in need of catabolic treatment may be advised to fast for two or three days, in order to cleanse the body, or perhaps to follow a light diet. A fast will then be followed by a program of constructive nutrition, including herbs to encourage cleansing and renourishing, together with hydrotherapy, breathing and exercises. It is very unlikely that you would be asked to fast during pregnancy, since fasting then is generally not advisable. Alternatively, treatment may be anabolic, which means, literally, "building up." This is best suited to weak patients who will benefit from supplements of certain minerals and vitamins.

As well as diet, the naturopath may also give advice on other "natural" treatments. These may include an exercise regime, taking fresh air, herbal cures and homeopathic medicines.

What You Can Do at Home

Most of what your therapist recommends can—and should—be carried out by you in your own home. To this extent, a naturopath is really a teacher more than a doctor. Naturopathy is more a way of life than a complementary therapy, helping you to help yourself:

- You may, for example, be advised to make certain changes in your diet; for example, eating more raw foods, more salads and more fresh fruit. You may also be told to avoid caffeine in coffee, tea and chocolate.
- You may be advised to give up smoking and to change your drinking habits.
- If you are suffering from an allergy, you may be advised to avoid certain foods most often wheat and dairy products.
- You may also be advised to take certain water treatments. These include saunas and steam baths, as well as baths using Epsom salts, oatmeal, seaweed or mud—all of which can help with certain skin conditions. Alternating hot and cold baths, hot or cold foot baths, hot and cold compresses which encourage the circulation and stimulate skin reflexes are also recommended. Water sprays which stimulate skin function, friction rubs with sea salt which stimulate skin function and encourage the circulation are also part of the naturopathic regime.

You may be advised to see your practitioner regularly during the first few weeks of home treatment, just to check on progress. After that, however, you will probably not need to see your therapist so often. This is, to a large extent, the beauty of naturopathy. What may have started as a professional therapy in response to ill-health, or a generalized fatigue which so many women experience during pregnancy, can soon become a way of maintaining good health for your family for life.

Herbalism

There are hundreds of plants, according to an ancient and worldwide system of medicine, that can be used to prevent and cure disease. Many of these can be used to alleviate some of the more common problems associated with pregnancy and to prepare you for the birth. The practice of herbal medicine uses plants—their roots, leaves, stems and seeds—prepared in a number of different ways to support the system and nurture it back to health. They can be taken internally in the form of teas, tinctures or as tablets or capsules; they can be applied externally in the form of an oil, an herbal bath or a hand or foot bath; or they can be applied directly to the skin in the form of a poultice, lotion or ointment. In many cases, herbs can provide a safe, natural and gentle alternative to drugs.

Herbal medicines have been used throughout the world for many thousands of years. In modern times, they have been the subject of much scientific investigation, which has revealed, in many cases, the pharmacological explanations for their uses. By a combination of ancient tradition and modern science, it has been established that many herbal remedies are not only effective but also safe for most of us to use.

The most valuable aspect of herbal remedies for most people is their application to everyday disorders. Complaints that respond most commonly to herbal medicine include coughs and colds, rhinitis, menstrual and pregnancy problems, all kinds of aches and pains, including headaches, toothache, earache and rheumatism, thrush, insomnia, skin conditions such as dandruff and acne, digestive problems such as diarrhea and constipation, nervous disorders, and many minor injuries including burns, scalds, cuts, bruises and insect bites. Herbal remedies are also used with considerable success as preventive medicines.

Its Role in Pregnancy

Herbal remedies have been used in pregnancy, as a preparation for childbirth and during labor itself all over the world for centuries and they are still in use today. Increasingly, women use herbs during pregnancy to enhance their general health, as well as to treat any problems that arise during pregnancy and to help ensure a safe and easy childbirth. By adopting a more natural approach to pregnancy and childbirth, they are taking more responsibility for themselves and relying less on an over-technological approach to childbirth. There are many different herbal remedies that can be used for various problems that commonly arise in pregnancy.

Herbs to Avoid in Pregnancy

Generally, herbal remedies are perfectly safe during all stages of pregnancy. There are certain herbs that should never be used in pregnancy as they can cause contractions of the uterus and may therefore threaten miscarriage. However, these are often helpful as the birth approaches and can be used to stimulate contractions during childbirth.

Herbs to Avoid

The following should all be avoided during pregnancy:

arbor vitae, autumn crocus, barberry, black cohosh, bloodroot, blue cohosh, broom, Chinese angelica, cotton root, feverfew, goldenseal, greater celandine, juniper, life root, male fern, mistletoe, mugwort, nutmeg (in large quantities), pennyroyal, poke root, rue, southernwood, tansy, thuja and wormwood

---

Preparing Herbal Remedies

There are a number of ways in which you can take herbal remedies either internally or externally.

Internal Uses

Infusions are made from the soft parts of the plant, such as the leaves, flowers and stems. They are prepared in the same way as a cup or pot of tea. The herbs are placed in a cup or a teapot and boiling water is poured over them to draw out the medicinal constituents of the plant. The mixture is covered and left to infuse for 10–15 minutes before it is drunk.

If you are using dried herbs, the standard dose is 25g (1oz) to 500ml (1 pint) of water. If you use fresh herbs, use two or three times the amount of herb to accommodate the extra water content of the plant. About 8oz (roughly a cupful) of the infusion can be taken three times daily for chronic problems or a cupful six times daily for more acute problems unless otherwise specified.

Herbs can be used singly or you can make up mixtures to suit your tastes. Many teabags of these aromatic herbs are sold in health food stores, and can be drunk daily as a healthy substitute for ordinary tea and coffee, which are best avoided during pregnancy. You can also make your own teabags using small muslin bags.

Decoctions are made from the harder, woody parts of plants, such as the bark, wood, roots, nuts and seeds. The pieces are first broken up into tiny pieces or powdered so that the medicinal value can be more easily extracted by the water. The plant material is placed in either a stainless steel or enamel saucepan. (Avoid aluminium pans, since aluminium is a soft metal which may combine chemically with the herbs and pollute your decoction or infusion.) Cold water is then poured over the herbs in the ratio of 25g (1oz) per 225ml (8fl oz), or roughly a cupful, of water plus a little more water to make up for any lost in the process. Cover and bring the mixture to the boil, then simmer for about 10 minutes. In this way, the greater heat of boiling acts to break down the herbs so that they release their essences into the water. Decoctions are used in the same dosages as infusions.

Tinctures are quite concentrated herbal medicines made using water and alcohol to extract the constituents, as well as to preserve the preparation almost indefinitely once made. If you visit a herbal practitioner, you are most likely to be given your herbs in tincture form. The advantage of using tinctures is that they are easily administered and stored, and you only have to take small amounts at a time—which is especially attractive to those people who dislike some of the stronger-tasting remedies. The usual dose is 1 teaspoon three times daily for chronic problems and 1 teaspoon six times daily for more acute cases. You can get tinctures from some health food stores.

External Uses

Herbal remedies can be used externally since many of their constituents are able to penetrate through the skin.

Herbal Baths can be taken to pamper yourself and still treat yourself medicinally. A few drops (between 4 and 6) of essential oil can be added to the bath water after it has been drawn; disperse the oils well before you get into the bath. Please check the *Aromatherapy* section for essential oils contraindicated during pregnancy (*see page 43*). The oils are carried on the steam and breathed in through the nose as well as being absorbed through the skin.

Alternatively, you can fill a small muslin bag with a mixture of fresh aromatic herbs and place it under the hot tap as you fill the bath, or pour 500ml (1 pint) or so of herbal infusion or decoction into your bath water. Again, check that the herbs you wish to use are safe to do so during pregnancy (*see the box on pages 25–27*).

Hand and foot baths have also been used for generations to treat a wide variety of problems. Infusions, decoctions, oils or herbs can be added to a bowl of warm water in which you immerse your feet for 8–10 minutes in the morning and your hands for the same length of time in the evening. The hands and feet are especially sensitive parts

of the body, through which the medicinal qualities of the plants pass easily, to be absorbed into the bloodstream. Sitz baths, too, may prove to be beneficial.

Ointments and Creams are suitable for certain conditions, such as varicose veins and piles, and to prevent stretch marks. They can be bought from health food stores or you can prepare them yourself.

Macerate 350g (12oz) of fresh or dried herbs in a mixture of about 480ml (16fl oz) of pure olive oil and 50g (2oz) of beeswax. Leave on a low heat for a few hours in a double boiler, until the medicinal constituents of the plant have been taken up by the oil. This mixture can then be strained through muslin and the herbs discarded. Pour into pots to cool and solidify.

Creams can also be prepared simply by mixing a few drops of essential oil or herbal tincture into aqueous cream which you can get from your local pharmacy.

Compresses are clean cloths wrung out in a hot or cold herbal infusion or decoction, then applied repeatedly, for as long as is necessary, to affected areas such as painful and engorged breasts, to reduce congestion and swelling.

Poultices are another useful form of external administration using the fresh or dried plant. The fresh herb needs to be bruised, and the dried herb needs to be powdered and mixed with water to form a paste. It is then applied to the affected part and bound with a light cotton bandage, which can be covered with plastic wrap to avoid staining clothes, and kept warm with a hot-water bottle. A hot bran poultice is particularly good to relieve mastitis.

Herbal Remedies for Conditions During Pregnancy

Problem	Recommended Herb	Method of Application
Infertility caused by hormonal imbalance	Vitex agnus castus (chaste tree or hemp tree), false unicorn root, wild yam and Chinese angelica	*Internally* Decoction or infusion from single herb or combination; drink a cupful three times daily Tincture; 1 teaspoon three times daily
Threatened miscarriage, with cramping pains in the stomach and bleeding*	False unicorn root, wild yam, black haw, cramp bark, raspberry leaves and squaw vine	*Internally* Decoction from either single herb or combination; sip a cupful every 15–60 minutes
Anemia	Comfrey leaves, burdock leaves, gentian, yellow dock root, raspberry leaves, centaury, hawthorn, rosehips, hops, skullcap, vervain	*Internally* Decoction or infusion from single herb or combination; drink a cupful three times daily
	Dandelion leaves, chives, nettles, elderberries, chickweed, sorrel, coriander leaves	*Internally* Add fresh to salads, soups, desserts
Backache	Ginger, cinnamon, lavender, rosemary	*Externally* Herbal baths; pour 500ml–1 litre (1–2 pints) of herbal decoction into a warm bath
Cystitis	Marshmallow, couch grass rhizomes, horsetail, chamomile, corn silk, buchu, echinacea, raspberry leaves	*Internally* Infusion or decoction from single herb or combination; drink a lukewarm or cold cupful every 20 minutes
Constipation	Burdock, yellow dock root, fennel, raspberry leaves, dandelion root, flaxseed, psyllium seeds (note: psyllium should be sprinkled into a cold liquid, stirred and drunk quickly)	*Internally* Infusion or decoction from single herb or combination (except psyllium seeds); drink a cupful one to three times daily Tincture; 1 teaspoon
	Lavender, lemon balm, peppermint, chamomile	*Externally* Herbal baths; pour 500ml–1 litre (1–2 pints) of decoction into a warm bath
Cramp	Horsetail, comfrey leaf, nettles, kelp, meadowsweet, wild oats, cramp bark, hawthorn leaves, flowers and berries, ginger	*Internally* Infusion or decoction from single herb or combination; drink a cupful three times daily
Heartburn	Meadowsweet, chamomile, peppermint, lemon balm, ginger	*Internally* Infusion or decoction; slowly sip at least two cupfuls throughout the day

* Seek medical attention

Herbal Remedies for Conditions During Pregnancy (cont)

Problem	Recommended Herb	Method of Application
Heartburn (cont)	Slippery elm	**Internally** Make a gruel and eat before each meal or take as tablets
	Gentian, marshmallow, peppermint, ginger, orange peel, tangerine peel, fennel, chamomile, dandelion root, licorice	**Internally** Decoction or infusion from single herb or combination; a cupful one to three times daily Dilute tincture; one teaspoon one to three times daily
High blood pressure*	Hawthorn flowers, leaves and berries, lime flowers, passion flower, cramp bark, yarrow	**Internally** Infusion or decoction from single herb or combination; a cupful three times daily Tincture; 1 teaspoon in a little water, three times daily
Fluid retention	Corn silk, horsetail, dandelion leaves, couch grass rhizomes, cleavers, plantain	**Internally** Infusion or decoction from single herb or combination; a cupful three times daily
Insomnia	Skullcap, passion flower, catnip, valerian, vervain, chamomile, lavender, lemon balm, raspberry leaves, lime flowers	**Internally** Infusion or decoction from single herb or combination; a cupful at night Tincture; 1–2 teaspoons at night
Mastitis*	Bran	**Externally** Hot poultice applied to breasts
Morning sickness	Lemon balm, hops, lavender flowers, chamomile flowers, wild yam, red raspberry leaves, gentian, peppermint leaves, verbena, meadowsweet, fennel seeds, ginger root, cinnamon bark, black horehound	**Internally** Infusion or decoction from single herb or combination; sip frequently throughout the day. Tincture; a few drops in a little water
Hemorrhoids	Comfrey leaf, catnip, calendula, bistort, witch hazel bark, oak bark, mullein leaves, horsetail, plantain, elderberry bark, beth root, lady's mantle	**Externally** Strong tea or 1 teaspoon of tincture in a little water. Soak wash cloth in mixture and use as compress; apply two or three times daily or more often as desired
	St John's wort, dandelion root, yellow dock root, cleavers, licorice, nettles	**Internally** Infusion or decoction from single herb or combination; a cupful three times daily
	Distilled witch hazel, pilewort ointment	**Externally** Apply directly two or three times daily

* Seek medical attention

Herbal Remedies for Conditions During Pregnancy (cont)

Problem	Recommended Herb	Method of Application
Stretch marks	Calendula, lavender flowers	**Externally** Soak flowers in wheat germ oil for two weeks and strain; apply oil daily
	Horsetail, raspberry leaves, corn silk, chickweed, kelp	**Internally** Infusion or decoction from single herb or combination; a cupful one to three times daily
Thrush	Calendula, rosemary, oregano, thyme, fennel seed, chamomile, American cranesbill, beth root, echinacea, cleavers, wild indigo	**Externally** Infusion or tincture; hold herb-soaked pads to vulva; bathe the affected area frequently with infusion or tincture; add infusion or tincture to sitz bath
	Thyme, echinacea, cleavers, chamomile, wild indigo, beth root	**Internally** Infusion or decoction from single herb or combination; a cupful one to three times daily
Varicose veins	Calendula, rosewater, oak bark, comfrey, plantain leaves, elderflowers	**Externally** Steep in or combine with a cupful of distilled witch hazel for an hour, then apply with wash cloth or cotton wool to areas affected two or three times daily
	Cleavers, yarrow, St John's wort, stone root, shepherd's purse, bistort root, peppermint	**Internally** Infusion or decoction from single herb or combination; a wineglassful two or three times daily. Tincture; 1 teaspoon in a little water, two or three times daily

The Consultation

At your first consultation, the medical herbalist will take a full case history, including details of your present condition and factors affecting your general health. The herbalist will want to know your menstrual and reproductive history, any previous illnesses, past drug therapy, inoculations and any reactions to them, allergies, any family tendencies to disease, trips overseas, stresses in your life, general energy levels and emotional state, your diet and lifestyle. The herbalist will also examine you.

Having established a clear picture of the whole person, the herbalist will prescribe plant remedies, as well as recommending changes in diet and lifestyle including exercise, relaxation and referrals if necessary. Counseling is often very much part of the consultation.

What You Can Do at Home

There are many over-the-counter herbal remedies and herbal medicine is one of the easiest of the natural therapies to use during your pregnancy.

Homeopathy

Homeopathy is a complementary therapy which concentrates on all aspects of a person—mental, emotional, spiritual and physical—and not just on the specific ailment. It is a complex system which aims to restore the body's natural balance and to strengthen its natural resistance to disease. Homeopathy was devised in 1796 by a German physician Samuel Hahnemann, as an alternative to the conventional practices of the day, such as bloodletting and purging, which he considered to be too harsh and too dangerous. Hahnemann believed that small doses were better than large ones and devised a system of diluting doses to the maximum degree.

Homeopathic remedies are all made from naturally occurring substances, such as plants, minerals, animals and, in some cases, diseased products. Remedies come in different potencies, as well as being in liquid, powder or pill form. The form most commonly available from pharmacies and health food stores are tablets in the 6 and 30 potencies. The higher the number, the greater the dilution and, according to Hahnemann, the greater the strength.

Its Role in Pregnancy

Homeopathic remedies are perfectly safe to take during pregnancy and, if used correctly, do not have any side-effects. But the ideal time to receive homeopathic treatment is before conception, when both partners should be treated. This raises your level of health, strengthens the immune system and increases your chances of conception, as well as preparing you for a healthy pregnancy.

Both preconceptually and throughout the pregnancy, you can benefit from good "constitutional" treatment which aims to treat your individual constitution rather than any specific condition or ailment. Constitutional treatment will help keep you and your baby healthy throughout your pregnancy, which should, in turn, assure you of the birth of a healthy baby.

One of homeopathy's great strengths is that it can help eradicate familial tendencies to illness. For example, if you or your partner suffers from eczema, your child stands a higher than average chance of suffering from it too. Treatment that is based on the parents' combined health, and that of both families, can deeply affect the health of your unborn child and can lessen this possibility.

Homeopathy is useful at all stages of pregnancy and many pregnant women visit their homeopath once a month. It is helpful in treating morning sickness and cramps, it can prevent constipation, and it can help with the labor as well as assisting in healing after birth. It relieves postnatal depression and has saved many mothers with engorged breasts from abandoning the struggle to breastfeed.

The Consultation

The principal aim of the homeopathic consultation is to find out what kind of person you are. The homeopath will obviously want to know about your physical discomforts but will also need to know how they affect you emotionally—whether they make you feel weepy or irritable, say—which will determine the remedy most suitable for you. The homeopath will ask you a myriad of questions about yourself, some of which may seem strange to you. You may be asked about your likes and dislikes in food, drink and climate, whether you like company or prefer to be alone, whether you sweat, what anxieties or fears you have, and how well or badly you sleep. The answers to all these questions will help the practitioner build up a picture of you and your lifestyle, which lead to a diagnosis and, in turn, will be matched to a remedy. The practitioner will then suggest a remedy or remedies for you to take at home.

Two consultations may be enough, but it is not uncommon for follow-up visits to be necessary—and possibly for quite some time if the condition is a chronic one—though patients tend to come less often as they begin to feel better. Homeopathy is not a licensed profession in the United States, but growing numbers of physicians, chiropractors and other health professionals are incorporating homeopathy into their practices. Naturopaths receive training in homeopathy, but other health professionals must seek out their own training. Homeopathic remedies are available in health food stores and many pharmacies; they rarely have side effects and can be self-prescribed by knowledgeable consumers.

Taking Remedies

There are particular ways in which remedies are taken; it is advisable that you wait at least 15 minutes before or after eating or drinking before taking a remedy. Tip the tablet on to your palm and put it under your tongue to dissolve.

Certain substances can stop remedies working, so they should be avoided while you are under treatment. These include mint in all its forms, including toothpaste (fennel toothpaste, available in health food stores, is a good alternative), tea, sweets, chewing gum, coffee, menthol, camphor and eucalyptus.

What You Can Do at Home

It is best to be treated professionally, but on occasions self-prescribing can be helpful keeping in mind some simple guidelines, which should help. Wherever possible, match your emotional and physical state to the remedy, and only take one remedy at a time. The exception to this is the use of Tissue Salts (see pages 31–32), which can be taken at the same time as another remedy.

The chart given on the following two pages forms a useful guide to the homeopathic remedies suitable for use during pregnancy. Remedies are given for many of the common conditions and complaints experienced by pregnant women; and there are also remedies that can help during labor and after giving birth.

As mentioned earlier, remedies come in different strengths and the higher the number, the greater the dilution and the greater the strength of the remedy. The 6 potency can be repeated hourly for up to six doses

Homeopathic Remedies for Pregnancy

Condition	Symptoms	Remedy
Constipation	Frequent unsuccessful urge to pass a stool	*Nux vomica*
Cystitis	Burning pain during and after urinating	*Cantharis*
	Frequent urge to pass urine, aggravated by stuffy room, fatty foods or emotional upsets. Clingy and weepy	*Pulsatilla*
	Prolapsed uterus, incontinence and irritability, all improved by exercise	*Sepia*
	Brought on by increased sexual activity	*Staphysagria*
Hemorrhage	Sudden red blood with fear of losing baby	*Aconite*
	Blood loss accompanied by great exhaustion	*China*
	Profuse bleeding with nausea and vomiting	*Ipecacuanha*
	Free-flowing clots, made worse by movement, and shooting pains in the vagina	*Sabina*
	Blood loss from injury	*Arnica*
Morning sickness	Crave food but feel nauseous when food is smelled	*Colchicum*
	Nausea is worse after vomiting	*Ipecacuanha*
	Vomiting frothy watery mucus, especially in the late morning. A craving for salt	*Natrum mur*
	Nausea worse at smell of food. Vomiting. Irritable. Worse in afternoon. Better on exercise and when keeping busy	*Sepia*
Cracked nipples	Sore cracked nipples	*Castor equus*
Engorged breasts	Hot, throbbing, red-streaked breasts	*Belladonna*
	Hard breasts, worse when any pressure is applied, and on movement *	*Bryonia*
	Hard, sensitive breasts. Abscesses. Pains in the nipples radiating all over the body when the baby feeds. *	*Phytollaca*
Labor	Weakness, exhaustion and labor not proceeding	*Caulophyllum*

* Seek medical attention

Homeopathic Remedies for Pregnancy (cont)

Condition	Symptoms	Remedy
Labor (cont)	Trembling and weakness	*Gelsemium*
	Weepy and indecisive, needing a lot of physical and emotional comfort	*Pulsatilla*
	Great fear and anxiety about labor	*Arsenicum album*
	Sudden fright and blood loss. Also useful for the baby if it is shaking and shocked at birth, and if it retains urine*	*Aconite*
	To help heal bruising	*Arnica*
Post-labor	To help heal soreness, especially if there has been a tear or an episiotomy	*Calendula*

* Seek medical attention

(*continued from page 29*)
and the 30 potency can be repeated every three hours for up to six doses. As soon as you start to feel any change, either physical or emotional, stop taking the remedy. This may be after just one dose or it may be after several. The reaction shows that the healing process has been triggered and will continue of its own accord. If you continue taking the remedy, the body will become over-stimulated and your symptoms may intensify. If there has been no change after six doses, however, you should seek professional help as you may not have chosen the correct remedy. Sometimes remedies can aggravate your symptoms temporarily. If this happens, stop taking the tablets and wait. After this initial intensification of symptoms, you should begin to feel better.

Please note that blood loss accompanied by exhaustion indicates a threat to a mother's life. So, if you experience these symptoms, do not hesitate to seek medical attention, and in the meantime treat with the appropriate homeopathic remedy which can help staunch the flow of blood.

Tissue Salts

There is a group of remedies called Tissue Salts, which are very helpful in pregnancy, both for you and for your baby. The body contains twelve vital mineral salts and, in pregnancy, their balance changes along with the growing needs of the fetus. They therefore need to be supplemented. The best way in which to do this is by taking Tissue Salts.

Five of the twelve Tissue Salts are particularly useful during pregnancy. They are: *Calc fluor* (Calcium fluoride), *Ferrum phos* (Iron phosphate) *Mag phos* (Magnesium phosphate), *Natrum mur* (Sodium chloride) and *Silica* (Silicon dioxide). A chart on the following page identifies each of these Tissue Salts, indicating the conditions they address, giving the correct dosage and suggesting the months of pregnancy during which you will find them most useful.

Choosing Your Tissue Salts

Tissue Salt	What It Does	Dose
Calc fluor	Prevents stretch marks and varicose veins. Good for tooth enamel	Take one twice a day throughout pregnancy
Ferrum phos	Strengthens blood vessels and arteries, and helps prevent anemia	Take one twice daily in months 2, 5, 6 and 9
Mag phos	Alleviates spasms and cramps	Take one twice daily in months 2, 3, 6 and 7
Natrum mur	Helps cope with metabolic changes of pregnancy. Prevents and cures dry skin, heartburn, swollen ankles and cravings for salty foods	Take one twice daily in months 3, 4, 7 and 8
Silica	Good for the blood, skin, hair and nails	Take one twice a day in months 4, 5, 8 and 9

Like regular homeopathic remedies, Tissue Salts are prepared in highly diluted dosages—usually with a 6 potency. They come in tablet form, which has a lactose base, and should be dissolved in the mouth rather than swallowed immediately.

Where to Buy Remedies

Homeopathic remedies and Tissue Salts can be bought at health food stores and most good pharmacies (*see page 157, Useful Addresses, for help with finding stockists*).

Tissue Salts Pregnancy Program

Month	Tissue Salt		
2	*Calc fluor*	*Mag phos*	*Ferrum phos*
3	*Calc fluor*	*Mag phos*	*Natrum mur*
4	*Calc fluor*	*Natrum mur*	*Silica*
5	*Calc fluor*	*Ferrum phos*	*Silica*
6	*Calc fluor*	*Mag phos*	*Ferrum phos*
7	*Calc fluor*	*Mag phos*	*Natrum mur*
8	*Calc fluor*	*Natrum mur*	*Silica*
9	*Calc fluor*	*Ferrum phos*	*Silica*

Massage

One of the most ancient complementary therapies, massage is found in every culture around the world. Perfectly suited to pregnancy, it soothes away aches and pains, and helps reduce tension. And the advantage of massage is that you and your partner can practice it together.

Touch is a very basic natural instinct and without it people can become bad-tempered and depressed. We all need to be encouraged to touch each other more, and massage, without any aggressive or sexual connotations, is the perfect way to do this. Even the simplest form of massage can be richly comforting, having a profoundly beneficial effect on your health. It improves circulation, it relaxes the muscles, it helps the digestion, it regulates the nervous system and it speeds up the elimination of waste products. These benefits, together with the psychological advantages of feeling pampered and cared for, soon produce a general feeling of profound well-being.

Massage is one of the oldest holistic therapies, taking into account a person's whole being—physical, mental and emotional. It is perhaps not surprising that Hippocrates, the ancient Greek physician hailed as the father of medicine, wrote as long ago as the fifth century BC: "The way to health is to have a scented bath and an oiled massage each day."

The main aim of massage is to relax both mind and body and thus relieve the stresses and strains of daily living. It is also successful in treating neck and back pain, particularly in people who spend the day hunched over a desk or sitting at the wheel of a car. Success has been claimed by therapists dealing with many other problems, including circulatory disorders, heart conditions, high blood pressure, headaches and insomnia, all of which can occur during pregnancy. Athletes and sports people can also gain enormously from massage, which eases stiffness and tones the muscles.

Its Role in Pregnancy

Gentle massage is highly beneficial to all pregnant women. Many practitioners are experienced in, and enjoy treating pregnant women, appreciating the tremendous benefits they are providing for them. Massage can also alleviate some of the most common, but minor, complaints of pregnancy. These include backache, insomnia, swollen legs and even morning sickness.

Back Massage

Backache is probably one of the most common complaints of pregnancy. Back massage can do a great deal to relieve this discomfort. As well as having a back massage done by a professional therapist, you can also ask your partner to do this for you. He should then use plenty of gentle stroking movements, which are very calming and should not apply deep pressure to the lower back, particularly during the first three months of pregnancy. These gentle strokes will help ease your backache, and give you a comforting sense of loving care being bestowed upon you, which is in itself deeply beneficial.

The Consultation

You may go to the therapist's consulting rooms or some therapists are happy to come to your home, particularly if you find it difficult to get around.

Massage is usually given in a warm, quiet room, with the person being massaged lying on a firm, comfortable surface—preferably on a special massage table. The practitioner will oil his or her hands, thus warming the oil before spreading it over the skin of the person being massaged. A light vegetable carrier oil scented with essential oils suitable for use during pregnancy (see page 48) may be chosen. The use of oil allows the therapist's hands to slide easily over the surface of the skin without unnecessary pulling, and the sensation of warm oil on the skin is very pleasant for the person being massaged.

The massage techniques in the West are based on Swedish massage, which relies on four basic massage movements. These are effleurage (stroking), petrissage (kneading), percussion (drumming) and friction (pressure). These four movements, used either singly or in combination, form the basis of any massage, though the individual practitioner will have favorite methods. A full-body massage usually lasts for about an hour, or an hour and a half if the face and head are included.

Never Massage When ...

Do not have a massage if you are suffering from any of the following:

any type of infection, for example colds or flu; a high temperature; acute back pain, especially when the pain shoots down the arms or legs; skin infection

---

Effleurage generally begins any massage and is useful for spreading oil evenly. It consists of slow, rhythmic stroking movements, covering a large area. Pressure should be firm as you stroke up the body (toward the heart) and more gentle as you stroke down.

Petrissage consists of grasping and squeezing handfuls of flesh or muscle, which are then kneaded like dough and released. Petrissage stimulates the circulation and helps to relax hard, contracted muscles.

Percussion involves short, fast, rhythmic movements, used mainly on large or fleshy areas. Percussion is generally inadvisable, other than on the legs, during pregnancy.

Friction is a series of small circular movements made by one or several fingers, the pads of the thumbs or heels of the hands. It stimulates circulation and helps keep the joints mobile.

What You Can Do at Home

Self-massage may not be as enjoyable as being massaged by someone else, but it can nevertheless be soothing and beneficial (see pages 37–41).

Positions for Massage

In early pregnancy it is still possible to lie on your front, perhaps placing a pillow under the chest if the breasts are tender. In later pregnancy, you can either straddle an upright chair sitting facing the back of it with a couple of pillows to lean against, or you can lie on your side with plenty of pillows for support.

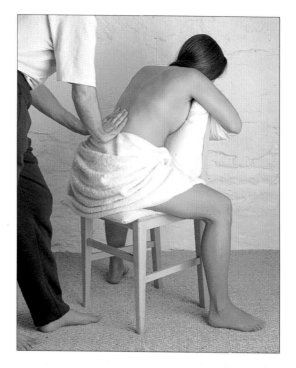

Right. Use a high-backed chair with pillows against the top and back of it so that you can lean forward comfortably with your head relaxed. The lower back, shoulders and neck can be massaged in this position.

Below. Lie on your side with your lower leg nearly straight and your upper leg bent at the knee. Place a cushion under the bent knee for support. You may want a pillow under your stomach also, and a couple of pillows or cushions supporting the upper body.

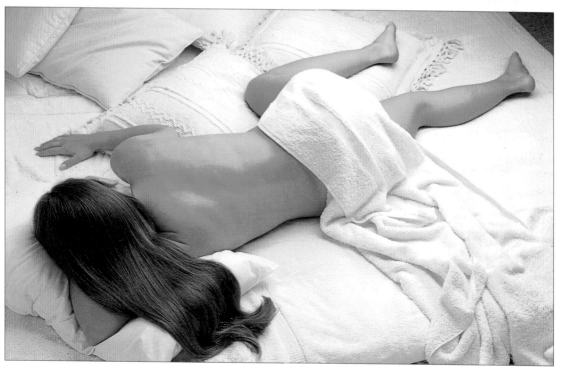

Right. *To effleurage the back, begin with your hands either side of the lower spine. Using the flats of your palms, glide up the back smoothly toward the shoulders. Then glide across the top of the shoulders and back down the sides of the body. Repeat, covering the whole back.*

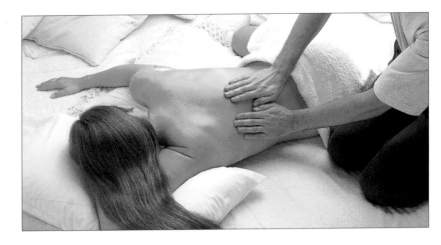

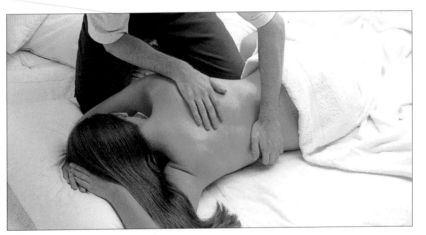

Left. *This petrissage stroke is working on the long muscles of the back. Kneeling opposite your partner, use the heel of your hand to gently push away from the spine and over the ribs. Work all the way along one side of the back from the bottom to just below the shoulder blades. Then swap sides to massage the other side.*

Right. *Finger circling or friction is shown here around the shoulder blades. Move the tips of your fingers in small circles, pressing quite firmly, all over the shoulder. Make sure the fingers are actually moving on the skin's surface as you do this. It is vital that your nails are fairly short to perform this stroke.*

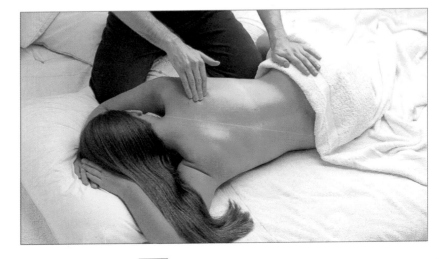

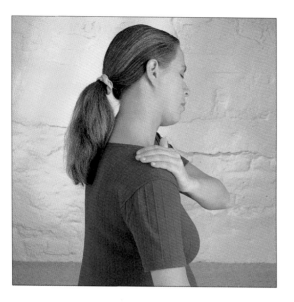

Shoulders

Tension tends to accumulate in the shoulders, causing aching shoulders, stiff necks and headaches. The shoulders are therefore a good place to begin your self-massage. You can use it to energize yourself before an appointment during the day or to unwind in the evening before going to bed. You can massage yourself while clothed or, if you prefer, unclothed using a vegetable oil.

1 *Stroke your right shoulder with your left hand. Stroke down the side of your neck, over your shoulder and down the arm to your elbow (left). Repeat this sequence at least three times, then do the same massage on the other shoulder.*

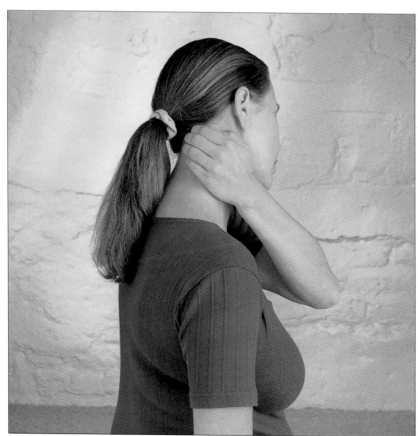

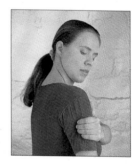

2 *Knead your shoulder with the opposite hand (above). Squeeze and release the flesh on your shoulder and at the top of your arm. Repeat several times on each shoulder.*

3 *Using your fingertips, make small circular movements on either side of the bones in your neck (left), pressing quite firmly. Work up the neck to the base of the skull.*

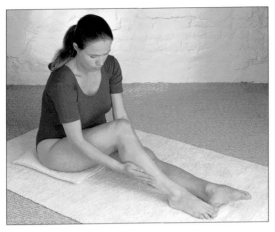

Legs

Massaging the legs is especially good if they ache. It stimulates the circulation and soothes tired or swollen legs. Avoid too much pressure on the inner leg area.

1 *Rest your foot on the floor and bend the knee (left). Using oil, stroke the whole leg from ankle to thigh quite firmly with both hands. Repeat this four or five times.*

2 *Knead the thigh and then the calf (see inset) using both hands alternately to squeeze and release the flesh. Repeat two or three times and then stroke the whole leg.*

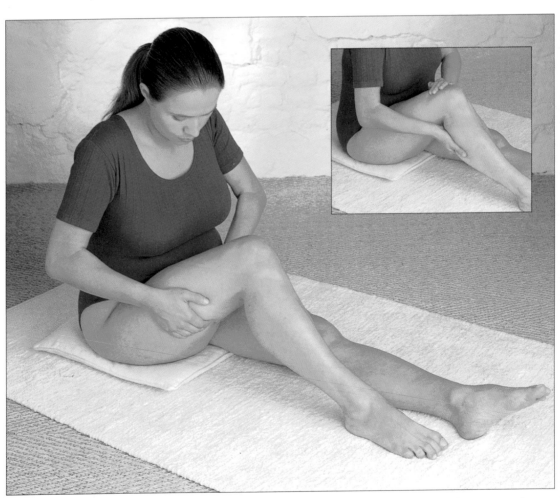

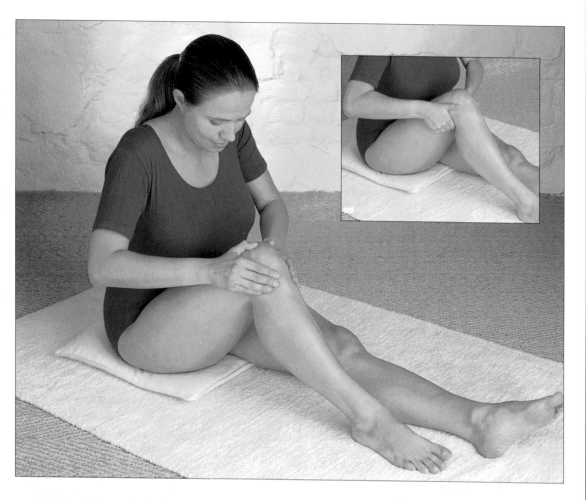

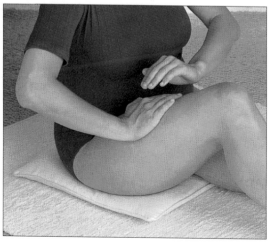

3 *Using your fingertips, stroke the area around the kneecap (above). Then stroke gently behind the knee up toward your thigh (see inset). Keep the strokes continually smooth and flowing.*

4 *Stroke the thigh firmly, working up the thigh from the knee using both hands, with one hand following the other (left). You will enjoy these smooth flowing strokes after the more energetic kneading.*

Now repeat steps 1–4 on the other leg.

Face

A face and scalp massage can get rid of headaches, as well as relieving fatigue and anxiety. Use a good quality face oil, or cream, to prevent dragging the skin.

1 *Put your hands over your face, with your fingers on the forehead and heels of the hands on the chin. Leave the hands quite still for a minute or two, then slowly draw them out toward your ears (below). Feel the tension easing away as you repeat the stroke.*

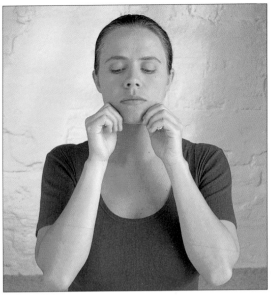

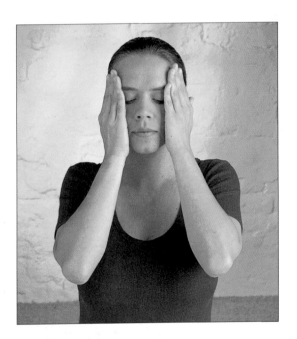

2 *Pinch along your jawline using the thumbs and knuckles of your forefingers (above). Begin just underneath the chin and work out gradually toward the ears. Pinch near the bone so that you are not stretching the skin. Repeat as many times as you like.*

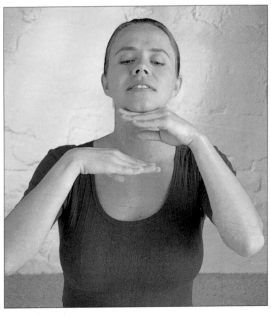

3 *Raise your head slightly and keep your jaw together so that your teeth do not bang against each other as you perform this movement. With the backs of your hands, and using each hand alternately, slap them gently and rhythmically under your chin (right). This is a pleasantly stimulating movement that will also help prevent a double chin. Repeat as many times as you like.*

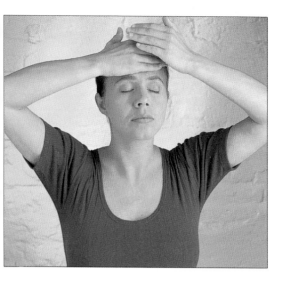

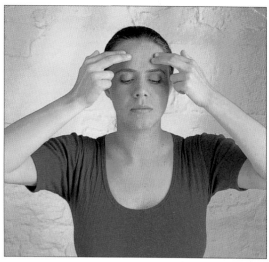

4 *Stroke your hands, one after the other, up your forehead, working from the bridge of the nose to the hairline. Close your eyes as you do this and repeat as often as you like. Then go on to massage your whole scalp, using claw-like movements with your fingertips.*

6 *Using the fingertips of your index and middle fingers, massage the entire forehead by making small circular movements all over this area. Press firmly but be careful not to drag the skin. Repeat as many times as you like.*

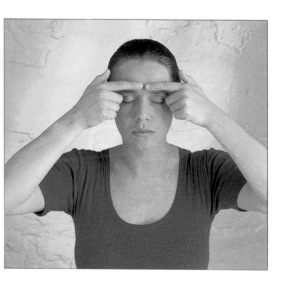

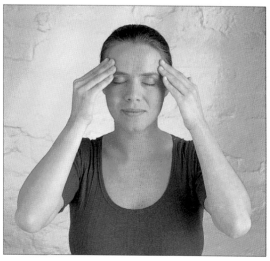

5 *Place both index fingers on the bridge of your nose and stroke firmly, first upward, and then across. This will help to reduce any frown lines and relieve tension. Repeat as many times as you like.*

7 *Using your fingertips, stroke your forehead gently, working from the center of the forehead toward your temples. Finally, press firmly against your temples and then release.*

Aromatherapy

Aromatherapy is a form of treatment which employs essential oils to treat a variety of conditions. These essential oils, as they are called, are extracted from various parts of plants. The oils are removed from the plant by complex extraction processes which retain all the important properties of the essential oil. These essential oils are then absorbed by the body, where their medicinal properties can help the body heal itself. Essential oils are absorbed by the body in a variety of ways; the main avenue is through the skin during massage, but they can also be inhaled, added to baths or used in compresses. In these ways, they are absorbed into the body fluids and bloodstream and can then set to work internally. When using essential oils for massage, the oils are always diluted in a carrier oil, and during pregnancy the recommended dilution is 0.5 to 1 percent (or 5 drops of essential oil to 2 tablespoons of carrier oil).

The history of essential oils is long and distinguished. They were particularly important to the ancient Egyptians. When Tutankhamun's tomb was opened in 1922, a great many scent pots were discovered, indicating that aromatherapy (although it was not called that) was widely used by the wealthy people of the time. The Greeks and Romans also used plant oils to heal wounds and to lessen inflammation.

In Europe, the effects of plants on the human body were first investigated in the sixteenth century. It became such a fashionable practice that by the end of the eighteenth century, essential oils were widely used in medicine. Interest in their use declined in the nineteenth century, when this practice was regarded as strange and somewhat eccentric, but was revived in the early part of this century by a French scientist called Gattefossé. Having burned his hand while conducting an experiment, he doused it in a dish of lavender oil which happened to be nearby. He was astounded by the speed with which his hand healed, and interest in the healing powers of plants was thus revived. It was Gattefossé who first coined the name "aromatherapy" in the 1920s.

Aromatherapy is believed to be most helpful in treating long-term conditions or recurring illnesses. Success has been claimed in treating stress and many stress-related problems including depression, headaches and insomnia. It has also been used to treat pain-related problems, such as arthritis and cramp, and skin problems such as eczema and acne.

Orthodox medics have become increasingly aware of the benefits to be gained from aromatherapy and scientific scrutiny has verified that many plants do indeed have medicinal properties. They have proved, too, that the scents of the oils affect cells in the nose, which in turn send messages to the brain. There is also strong evidence that the oils do indeed penetrate the skin. Further research is being done to find out exactly how aromatherapy works.

Its Role in Pregnancy

The main and immediate effect of aromatherapy is relaxation, which is very beneficial in pregnancy. It has a number of other benefits, including: promoting a feeling of well-being; reducing fatigue; relieving backache; improving circulation and so reducing any tendency to varicose veins and hemorrhoids; helping counteract fluid retention; toning the muscles and so reducing aches and pains; maintaining the suppleness and elasticity of the skin which helps prevent stretch marks and preparing you for childbirth, both physically and emotionally.

Various oils can be used to treat many of the minor problems of pregnancy such as constipation, nausea, heartburn and so on. All essential oils that are used in pregnancy should be diluted 0.5 to 1 percent (more simply put, use 5 drops of essential oil to every 2 tablespoons of carrier oil) in a vegetable carrier oil such as jojoba, sesame or almond. However, it is important to exercise caution when using essential oils during pregnancy. To begin with you must tell your therapist that you are pregnant, even in the very early months. There are a number of essential oils which are not suitable for use during pregnancy, especially during the first three months; some oils are emmenagogues, which means they stimulate menstruation—something to be avoided in early pregnancy. It is especially important not to use any essential oils which have oxytocic properties which stimulate contractions of the uterus.

The Consultation

A consultation begins with a discussion of your general health and lifestyle. The aromatherapist will then select the oils that are deemed to be best for you, taking into account your personality, the nature of your problem and the fact that you are pregnant. A full aromatherapy massage takes about an hour and is deliciously luxurious and relaxing. The therapist will probably mix some oils for you to use at home, so you can continue the treatment yourself. They may also suggest that you would benefit from further professional treatments.

Oils to Avoid During Pregnancy

Angelica, basil, cedarwood, chamomile, cinnamon bark, clary sage, cypress, fennel, juniper, ginger, hyssop, marjoram, myrrh, nutmeg, oregano, parsley, peppermint, rose absolute, rose otto, rosemary, sage, savory, thyme

Many oils, particularly the citrus family of essential oils, are phototoxic and should therefore not be used before sunbathing. These oils can cause blotching on the skin if exposed to the sun and include:

tangerine, bergamot, fennel, mandarin, grapefruit, lemon, orange, lime

---

Aromatherapy Massage

The following three pages set out a relaxing aromatherapy massage. Make sure that the essential oils you mix with carrier oil are not included in the list above.

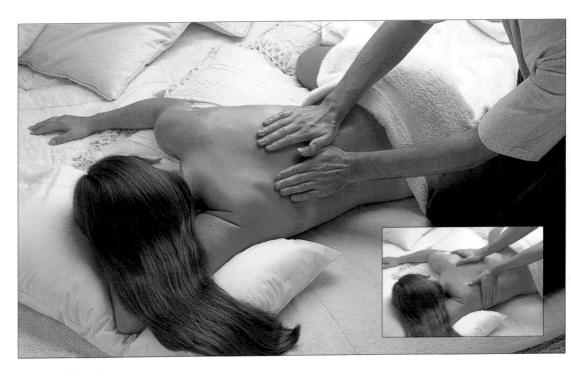

1 *With your partner lying on her front (above, see page 35), glide your hands up the back, out across the shoulders and back down the sides of the body (inset).*

2 *Work deeply into the shoulder by pushing the muscle forward over the shoulder, then lift and pull back (see left). Follow with your other hand, creating a "wringing" movement. Repeat several times on each shoulder.*

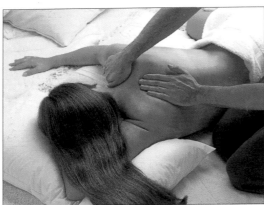

3 *The head should be leaning forward on the pillows if straddling a chair, or if lying face down place the hands under the forehead. Using one hand with thumb spread apart from fingers, glide up the neck using the inside edges of the thumb and index finger (see right). As you come to the top of the neck give a gentle squeeze. Be careful not to drag the skin or pull the hair of the neck. Repeat this movement squeezing gently.*

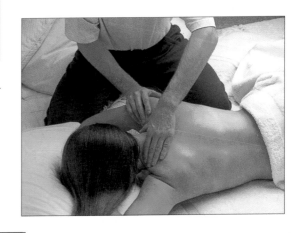

4 *In any of the suggested positions, including lying on the back as shown below, you can use your fingertips quite firmly to massage the scalp. You may want to remove any excess oil from your hands before you do this, alternatively you can use an oil to nourish your hair and scalp. Use a deep shampooing action that not only affects the scalp but works firmly into the head. Move both hands around the head, circling firmly over the back, sides and top of the head to the hairline. Finish by tugging gently at the roots of the hair.*

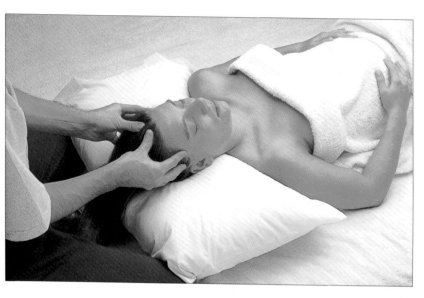

5 *Massage on the belly is best received while lying on your back. As your stomach gets bigger and bigger, lying flat on the back will become more uncomfortable, and you might find breathing normally a little difficult as well. Try supporting the head, shoulders and knees with pillows while lying down, so that you are almost in a sitting position (below).*

6 *Massage the belly with a gentle circling movement clockwise over the abdomen. Start with small clockwise circles, becoming larger as the belly grows. Using a good quality carrier oil and essential oils can help prevent stretch marks. As the baby grows, this is a wonderful massage as you feel the baby moving around under the hands. Let your hands slide under the back from time to time and give a gentle lift to the body to relieve strain on back muscles.*

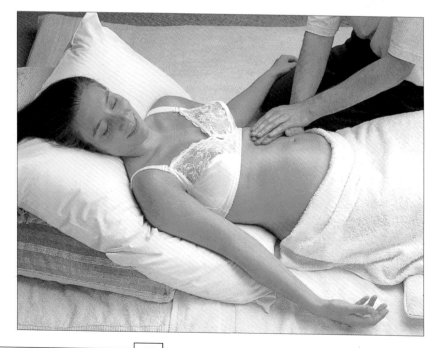

7 *The legs can also be massaged in this position. Bend the leg at the knee and sitting at your partner's foot, oil the hands and glide up the back of the leg over the calf to the knee with both hands flat (right). Stop behind the knee and repeat several times, again slight pressure on the way up, light contact on the way back. You can squeeze the muscles of the calf but beware of varicose veins and do not squeeze if these are present.*

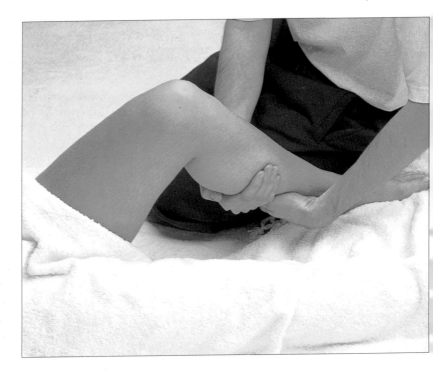

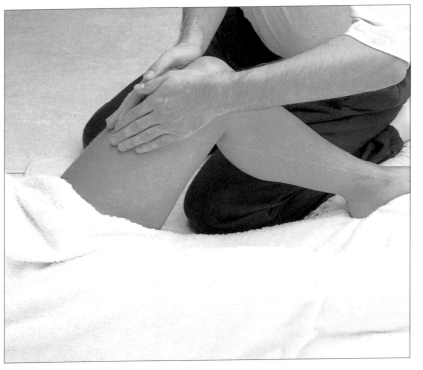

8 *For thigh massage, use both hands again to stroke from knee to groin area (left). Leave the knee bent to get to the back of the thigh. You may find it easier to use the knuckles in the hamstrings or straighten the leg and do several effleurage strokes over the thigh. Be careful not to apply pressure or too much squeezing to the inner leg area. Repeat for other leg.*

What You Can Do at Home

Aromatherapy is easy to practice at home and there are many short courses available which teach you the basic principles. There are several methods you can use to treat yourself. These include the following:

Baths for tension, backache, constipation, cystitis, aching muscles, insomnia, headaches, coughs and colds. Add 4–6 drops of essential oil, or a combination of several essential oils, to a hot bath , dispersing the oil well before you get in. If you have sensitive skin dilute the essential oil in a small amount of full fat milk or vegetable oil before adding to your bath. Lie back in the water, relax and breathe deeply. Stay in the bath for between 10 and 15 minutes.

Foot and Hand Baths for localized aches and pains, and swelling. Add 8–10 drops of essential oil to a large bowl of hand-hot water. Soak the feet or hands in the water for between 10 and 15 minutes, topping up with warm water if it gets cold. When you take your feet or hands out of the water, wrap them in a dry warm towel for a further 15 minutes.

Massage for stress, skin problems, skin complaints, cramps, fluid retention, breathing difficulties and to avoid stretch marks. Apply diluted essential oils to the skin and massage in following the massage sequence on pages 37–41 if you are massaging yourself, or pages 44–46 if your partner is massaging you. An essential oil should always be diluted in a vegetable carrier oil, such as jojoba, sesame or almond. As mentioned earlier, during pregnancy, essential oils should always be diluted by 0.5 to 1 percent in a carrier oil.

Compresses for bruises, varicose veins, hemorrhoids, sprains, burns and scalds. Add between 8–10 drops of essential oil to half a cup of water. Disperse well. Soak a piece of cotton wool in this, wring it out and place over the affected area. Place a warm towel over the compress and leave it in place for at least two hours.

Inhalation for tension, insomnia, nausea, breathing difficulties, coughs and colds. Put 1–2 drops of essential oil on to a tissue, a handkerchief or a kitchen towel and inhale. Place the tissue or handkerchief on your pillow at night if you are having problems breathing. A steam inhalation can be done by putting 5–10 drops of the essential oil into a bowl of hot water. Sit with your head above the bowl and cover both head and bowl with a towel to contain the vapor. Breathe deeply and close your eyes to prevent irritation.

Cautions

- *Do not take any essential oils orally.*
- *Use only those labelled "pure essential oil."*
- *Essential oils should be stored in dark bottles.*
- *Only lavender and tea tree oil may be used undiluted in small amounts.*
- *Generally, stimulating and emmenagogic essences should not be used in pregnancy.*
- *Avoid contact of oils with eyes and genitals, and breasts when breastfeeding.*
- *Keep oils away from light sources and out of the reach of children.*
- *Do not use certain essential oils if taking homeopathic remedies.*
- *Test essential oils by applying a few drops diluted in carrier oil to a fabric plaster and leave on for 24 hours or until any irritation occurs.*

Aromatherapy Oils and Their Therapeutic Uses

Essential Oil	Problem	Properties
Cajeput *Melaleuca leucodendron*	Breathing difficulties, indigestion, toothache, skin conditions, aches and pains, fatigue	Uplifting, soothing, antiseptic **Potential skin irritant**
Chamomile *Anthemis nobilis*	Nausea, heartburn, indigestion, depression, headache, fluid retention, cystitis, thrush, tension during labor	Refreshing, toning, relaxing, digestive, antiseptic, antifungal **To be avoided in the first three months of pregnancy**
Eucalyptus *Eucalyptus globulus*	Fluid retention, muscular pain, headaches, infections, breathing difficulties, fever, mastitis	Purifying, clears the air, antiseptic **Potential skin irritant**
Geranium *Pelargonium graveolens*	Cellulite, mastitis, premenstrual tension, diarrhea, stress, tension, skin conditions, improves circulation, fluid retention, tension during labor	Toning, refreshing, relaxing, antiseptic, antifungal **Do not use on breasts if breast-feeding as it can be over-stimulating for a young baby**
Lavender *Lavandula angustifolia;* *Lavandula officinalis*	Depression, indigestion, insomnia, anxiety, aches and pains, fatigue, infections, high blood pressure, burns, skin conditions, preventing stretch marks, tension during labor	Relaxing, refreshing, toning, antiseptic, antispasmodic, analgesic
Lemon *Citrus limon*	Circulatory problems, high blood pressure, skin conditions, infections	Toning, refreshing, fortifying, purifying, antiseptic **Potential skin irritant; phototoxic**
Neroli *Citrus aurantium*	Anxiety, stress, insomnia, skin conditions, preventing stretch marks	Relaxing, fortifying
Pine *Pinus sylvestris*	Infections, fluid retention, flu, coughs and colds, catarrhal congestion	Refreshing, soothing, antiseptic, expectorant, decongestant **Potential skin irritant**
Sandalwood *Santalum album*	Infections, fluid retention, skin conditions, respiratory infections	Soothing, refreshing, diuretic, stimulant, said to be an aphrodisiac
Tangerine *Citrus reticulata*	Aches and pains, fluid retention, excellent for preventing stretch marks, indigestion, constipation	Toning, soothing, refreshing, harmonizes body and mind **Potential skin irritant; phototoxic**

Acupuncture

Acupuncture is a system of medicine based on an ancient Chinese belief that the body is divided by invisible energy channels, called "meridians." Each of the meridians is said to be linked to a particular internal organ. Thus each organ of the body can be treated by stimulating the relevant meridian. Acupuncture uses needles as thin as a strand of hair to activate the body's energy channels in order to treat disease, to bolster the immune system, to promote the body's natural healing powers and to alleviate fatigue. Not only will you find acupuncture useful during your pregnancy, but you can also use it to provide effective pain relief during your labor.

This painless treatment involves inserting very fine hairlike needles into the skin in quite specific places known as acupuncture points which lie along the meridians. The needles have the effect of unblocking the flow of energy or life force (called *Qi* or *Ch'i*) which runs through the meridians. There are fourteen meridians in all, each of which is named after the organ that it represents.

Any disorder, whether physical or emotional, is believed to alter the flow of energy through the meridians. It can make it too slow, too fast or it can divert it to the wrong organ, or even block it completely. An acupuncturist aims to correct the flow and balance of energy—in other words, unblock it or make it flow faster or slower according to what is wrong with it—and cause it to return to its normal rate. When an organ is diseased, the corresponding acupuncture points often become tender. According to acupuncturists, the tenderness will disappear as soon as the disease is treated, whether it is treated by conventional medicine or by acupuncture.

Although acupuncture is an ancient Chinese therapy, it continues to play an integral part in modern Chinese medicine. It regards the body as a balance between the two opposing yet complementary natural forces known as *yin*, which is the female force, and *yang*, which is the male force. Yin is thought to be passive and peaceful while yang, on the other hand, is aggressive and confrontational. Yin represents dark, cold, moisture and swelling. Yang represents light, heat, dryness and tautness. According to Chinese medicine, it is an imbalance between yin and yang which cause diseases. Too much yin, for example, can cause dull pains, chills and fatigue. Too much yang can cause swelling, pain, headaches and high blood pressure.

The aim of acupuncture is to identify and treat any imbalance of yin and yang by inserting needles at the correct acupuncture points. According to ancient Chinese tradition, there are 365 acupuncture points, but the Chinese have now in fact described about 1000 points in all.

The concept that lies at the root of acupuncture, with its strange blend of physical and metaphysical interpretation, can be difficult for Westerners to understand. But it certainly does work. There is a wealth of evidence to suggest that acupuncture works for a great many people suffering from a great many different complaints. In the West, acupuncture is used mostly to treat painful conditions like back pain, arthritis and rheumatism. Research on the role of acupuncture in pain relief has shown that it can cause the body to produce natural pain-relieving substances, or opiates, known as *endorphins* and *enkephalins*, which dull the senses. Acupuncture has been used successfully to relieve pain during dentistry, surgery and childbirth.

Acupuncture has also been helpful to people suffering from many other complaints including allergies, asthma, heart conditions, digestive problems, insomnia, headache and migraine, anxiety, stress, fatigue, backache and back disorders, skin conditions and ulcers.

The Fourteen Meridians

The fourteen meridians correspond to particular organs in the body. These are the heart, small intestine, bladder, liver, gallbladder, kidneys, lungs, colon, stomach, spleen, pericardium, "triple heater," which controls the function of the endocrine glands (not recognized by Western medicine); "Ren" or "conception," which runs vertically up the center of the front of the body (not recognized by Western medicine) and "Du" or "governor," which runs vertically up the center of the back of the body (not recognized by Western medicine).

Its Role in Pregnancy

Before a woman can conceive, her body, according to Chinese beliefs, must be in perfect harmony. Only then can the flow of energy necessary for the formation of a healthy fetus be normal. Acupuncture is the key to obtaining that perfect balance. During pregnancy, too, the flow of energy through the body must be right in order for the fetus to develop in as healthy a way as possible. One of the most common complaints in pregnancy—morning sickness—can be greatly alleviated by acupuncture.

There are, however, certain points on each meridian that must be avoided during pregnancy. These points vary according to what stage of pregnancy you have reached. In general, they are the points that will stimulate the uterus, which is obviously not advisable in the early stages of pregnancy as it can lead to miscarriage.

However, it is in labor that acupuncture has claimed its greatest triumphs. There are many acupuncturists who specialize in treating pregnant women, and who are happy to go to the hospital with you to provide safe and natural pain relief. Many acupuncturists who attend births observe that a woman in labor who is being treated with acupuncture never panics and succeeds in giving birth in a relaxed and easy way.

Few hospitals—or physicians—in the US are prepared for deliveries to be accompanied by an acupuncturist; midwives may be more open-minded. Acupuncture can also be used to encourage the dilation of the cervix and to speed things along in labor—or slow it down, whichever is required.

The Consultation

The first thing an acupuncturist will do is to take a detailed case history, including asking you about your lifestyle, diet, exercise, sleep patterns and stress levels. The therapist will then diagnose any complaints according to the ancient rules of Chinese diagnosis. Your tongue, skin coloring and condition, hair, posture and general demeanor will all be examined, along with the sound of your breathing and your voice. Above all, though, the most important tool acupuncturists have is pulse diagnosis, which enables them to tell the state of energy in the meridians simply by taking your radial artery pulse at the wrist.

There are six pulses at each wrist, making twelve in all. Each pulse represents one of the twelve main organs and functions of the body. Taking the pulses is known as "palpating." The experienced acupuncturist can diagnose hundreds of different conditions by palpating. It is such a sensitive diagnostic tool, in fact, that it can tell the skilled practitioner about your past illnesses and warn about future illnesses.

Once diagnosis has been made, the acupuncturist will then carefully and painlessly insert needles into acupuncture points in the body. The needles are made of very fine stainless steel, and *must* be disposable, presented in sealed sterilized packs, thus eliminating any possibility of transferring infection, the most serious risks being AIDS or infectious hepatitis.

The insertion of the needles is usually quick, painless and bloodless. The acupuncturist inserts a number of hair-thin needles and then rotates them gently between finger and thumb to draw or disperse energy from a point. You will probably experience a slight numbness or tingling sensation.

The number of needles used varies. It can be as few as one or two, or as many as fifteen. Generally speaking, the more experienced the acupuncturist, the fewer the needles used. They can be left in for just a few minutes, or they can stay in for up to thirty minutes. This depends on the practitioner, the patient and the condition being treated.

You may feel an improvement within the first four or five visits. It would be a very lucky patient indeed for whom just one session was enough to cure any problem. Many patients report a feeling of lightness or buoyancy, or extreme relaxation, after treatment. A complex problem, such as asthma, may require more sessions before there is any noticeable improvement. If there is absolutely no improvement after about eight sessions, acupuncture may not be the answer for that particular patient or that particular complaint.

Occasionally, a patient may feel worse after the initial treatment. This is usually because the acupuncturist has overstimulated the body's energies, in which case fewer needles will probably be used, and for a shorter time, at the next session.

Many acupuncturists recommend a visit at each change of season—that is, four times a year to give the body an overall tune-up; a bit like having a car serviced regularly.

What You Can Do at Home

Acupuncture cannot be done at home—either by you or by your partner—unless, of course, he is an acupuncturist. Even acupuncturists rarely practice on themselves. Acupuncture must never be attempted by anyone who is not fully trained and qualified. In untrained hands, it can be dangerous.

Acupressure

This ancient massage technique, with a system of pressure points which correspond to acupuncture points, is something you and your partner can practice and enjoy at home. It is also ideal for those of us who are attracted by the theory of acupuncture but shy away from the prospect of needles.

We all use a form of acupressure when we rub a part of the body that hurts, or press our hands against our forehead to ease a headache. Acupressure is thought to be a forerunner of acupuncture, although it uses firm thumb or fingertip pressure rather than needles. Like acupuncture, it is used to balance the flow of *Ch'i*, or energy, through the meridians. There are various different schools of acupressure; the differences lie mainly in the chosen combinations of pressure points and in the degree of pressure applied.

Acupressure is largely a system of relieving symptoms rather than treating disease, though it is said to improve the body's own healing powers and thus to alleviate and prevent illness. It is thought to be particularly appropriate for people suffering from allergy, arthritis, asthma, back pain, circulatory problems, depression, digestive troubles, insomnia, migraine and stress.

Its Role in Pregnancy

As in acupuncture, there are some acupressure points that must not be worked on during pregnancy. It is important to tell your therapist that you are pregnant and to ask for specific advice for you as an individual. Only light pressure should be used on pregnant women, and, in general, the abdomen should be avoided, especially in the first three months of pregnancy.

The Consultation

All practitioners begin by taking a case history, including details of your lifestyle and diet. The therapist will also take your pulses, in much same way as in an acupuncture consultation. Pressure will then be applied to certain points, depending on whether the therapist wants to stimulate or sedate the energy channels. Pressure may be applied in a variety of different ways, using the thumbs, fingertips, palms, knees, elbows and even feet. Pain relief may be sudden, particularly for acute problems. Chronic conditions may take longer.

What You Can Do at Home

It is quite safe to use acupressure at home, particularly for common problems such as headache and nausea. A few sessions with a qualified therapist will teach you exactly what to do and what not to do, since there are some points that should never be stimulated in pregnancy. Overstimulation of certain points can occasionally cause a temporary worsening of symptoms. Although you can use acupressure on yourself, it is always better—not to say more pleasant—to get your partner to do it for you.

One particularly common complaint in pregnancy is morning sickness, which responds very well to acupressure. Make sure you are sitting comfortably and that you are warm. Then massage these points yourself, or get someone to do it for you. Press with your thumb on a point about 5cm (2in) from the wrist on the inside of the arm. Apply pressure for five to ten minutes. The pressure should cause some minor discomfort, but definitely not pain. Repeat the pressure as often as necessary.

Shiatsu

Shiatsu is the Japanese word for "finger pressure" and it has been practiced in the Far East for hundreds of years. Although similar to acupressure because it is based on pressure points along meridian lines associated with the function of the vital organs, shiatsu lays more emphasis on prevention of disease rather than treating symptoms. Again like acupressure, it aim is to stimulate *Ch'i* (*ki* in Japanese), which means "energy," but instead of stimulating energy to relieve pain, shiatsu places the emphasis on freeing energy channels to promote overall health. In Japan, the technique is considered to be a means of early diagnosis as well as a disease preventive, and many people undergo regular shiatsu treatment, sometimes as often as once a week. It is thought to benefit the body, mind, emotions and spirit at the same time. Shiatsu is considered to be particularly effective in treating migraine, back pain, toothache, digestive troubles, depression and insomnia, and in strengthening the immune system.

Its Role in Pregnancy

As in acupressure, there are certain points on each meridian that should be avoided during pregnancy. With this proviso, shiatsu can be beneficial throughout pregnancy because it strengthens the immune system at a time when many medicines are not recommended. It also aids relaxation and lifts the spirits.

Take particular care during the first three months of pregnancy, since this is the time when all the baby's organ systems are developing. Shiatsu should generally be kept simple and non-specific during this trimester—supportive rather than intrusive. During the second three months, shiatsu can become more specific, in order to deal with problems such as backache, constipation and hemorrhoids. A shiatsu practitioner can attend the birth to help with pain relief, or can teach the father some simple pain relief techniques to support the mother.

The Consultation

Unlike acupuncturists, practitioners of shiatsu use no special equipment; a firm surface, such as a carpeted floor, in a clean, warm, quiet room is all that is required. Treatment is available at therapy centers, and some practitioners will come to their clients' homes. You should wear loose clothes, which will be comfortable for you and facilitate the practitioner's touch.

The first session usually begins with the practitioner taking your case history. As in acupuncture, the therapist will take your pulses, of which there are six on each wrist, each associated with a vital organ.

The treatment is then somewhat like a massage, the only difference being that the therapist is working on pressure points along the meridians. You will spend some time on your back, some on your front, some sitting up. Shiatsu is not carried out in any set order.

Pressure is applied in many different ways and a series of different movements may be executed over a part of the body, rather than over one pressure point. Sometimes the bulb of the thumb is used, sometimes the fingers, sometimes the palm or the heel of the hand. An elbow may be used, or perhaps a forearm or a knee. How hard the therapist applies pressure depends on many things, including where it is to be applied, how you react and whether you require a tonifying or sedating effect. Pressure is applied for a few seconds at a time and is repeated several times at each spot. According to Namikoshi, who popularized the therapy half a century or so ago, the pressure should produce a sensation somewhere between pain and pleasure. A shiatsu session usually lasts about an hour.

What You Can Do at Home

Shiatsu developed as a home treatment handed down from one generation to another, and it is indeed possible to learn how to apply finger pressure at home. It is best to learn the techniques from a trained shiatsu practitioner, particularly if you are pregnant, when certain pressure points should be avoided. However, the following step-by-steps to relieve tired feet are perfectly safe.

Tired Feet

The shiatsu massage sequence, shown opposite, is a wonderful way to relieve tired and aching feet at the end of the day.

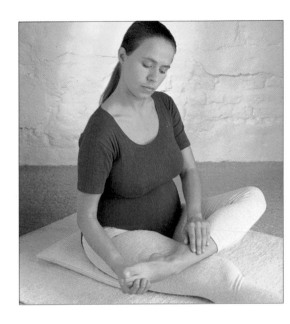

1 *Grasp the ball of your foot and make three slow rotations clockwise, then three counterclockwise.*

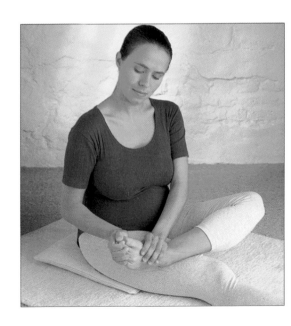

2 *Hold your toes in one hand and stabilize your foot with the other hand. Rotate all toes three times in each direction.*

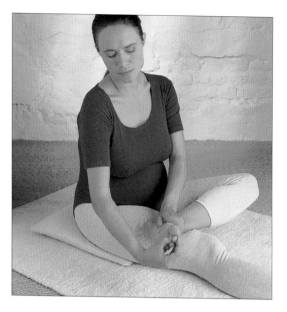

3 *Squeeze and massage each toe between your fingers, from its tip toward the foot.*

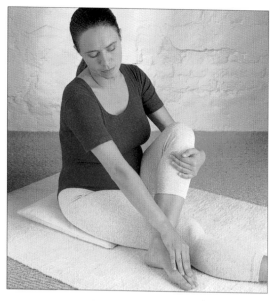

5 *Slide your fingers along the grooves on the top of your foot, from toes to ankle, several times.*

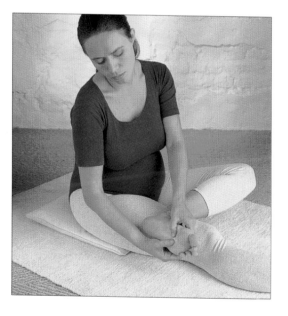

4 *Use both thumbs to massage the sole of your foot with small circular movements from heel to toes and across the instep and ball of your foot.*

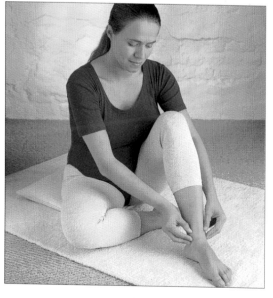

6 *Massage both ankle bones of the foot at the same time with your fingers and thumbs, using a circular massaging motion.*

Reflexology

Reflexology, which is also known as reflex zone therapy, is based on the principle that there are reflexes or energy channels in the feet which relate to every organ and function in the body. By applying pressure to these reflex points, the energy channels in these areas are opened, restoring the energy flow around the body to a healthy balance. Reflexologists regard the feet as a "mirror" of the body, with the left foot relating to the left-hand side of the body, and the right foot to the right-hand side. They believe that ill-health occurs when energy channels become blocked, causing particular areas of damage. Massage aims to break up those blockages, and allows the energy to flow again, so healing the damage.

Reflexology was practiced in China some 5000 years ago, and in ancient Egypt some 4000 years ago. It was rediscovered in 1913, by an American ear, nose and throat specialist, Dr William Fitzgerald. He found that when certain points on the feet were pressed, anesthesia was induced in specific parts of the body. Through experimentation in applying pressure to the feet, either with his hands or with special instruments, he evolved a healing system which he named zone therapy.

Complaints that have been treated successfully with reflexology include back pain, migraine, sinus problems, digestive troubles, arthritis, menstrual problems, infertility, anxiety and stress. Reflexologists also claim that they can sometimes predict a potential problem, and then take pre-emptive action to avoid the problem arising. Reflexology treatment can be very beneficial to the pregnant woman and is particularly helpful in alleviating some postnatal problems.

Its Role in Pregnancy

Reflexology is reported to help overcome fertility problems in both sexes but particularly those in women. Frequently, a woman who finds that she is unable to conceive, undergoes a series of gynecological tests. If nothing abnormal is found, she may be offered a fertility drug or told that nothing further can be done to help her. If told the latter, it can cause a great deal of stress and unhappiness.

The important role that reflexology can play in this situation lies in its power to alleviate stress and induce a deep sense of peace and relaxation. If a man is able to treat his partner, it will create a sense of closeness and warmth between them allowing the woman to be physically receptive. As well as working with any stress element, the endocrine glands and reproductive organs are gently stimulated during the treatment, helping to remove any energy blocks.

It is a surprisingly powerful form of therapy, which means that it is not always suitable in the first three months of pregnancy. An experienced practitioner will, however, be able to advise you. After the initial trimester of pregnancy, reflexology can help with relaxation and sleeping problems. It can also help to boost the immune system.

The Consultation

At the first visit, the reflexologist will take a detailed case history. You will then lie in a comfortable reclining position, with the feet raised, shoes and socks removed. The therapist will then examine your feet, noting their general appearance, temperature and color. Before treatment begins, the reflexologist will apply talcum powder to your feet to prevent their hands sticking to your feet, thereby allowing a smooth and even movement over the surface of your skin.

The therapist will use thumb pressure of varying strengths over pressure points in the feet, concentrating on any tender areas; these indicate parts of the body that are out of balance. Sessions last about fifty to sixty minutes, and may be weekly to start with, then may be at intervals of two or three weeks. During a course of treatment, the body goes through a process of detoxification, which may manifest itself in aching joints, diarrhea or increased urination. This does not always happen, but if it does, it should be regarded as a good sign and will not, in any case, last long.

What You Can Do at Home

During the first three months of pregnancy, it is advisable to attend a qualified reflexologist and not treat yourself, particularly if there is a history of miscarriage or if this is your first pregnancy. Reflexology is a holistic therapy, and as such the whole body should be treated, paying special attention to specific problems you may be suffering.

The best results are obtained through consultation with a qualified practitioner, though it is possible for you to treat some ailments yourself. Only minor complaints, including back and neck pain, tension, sinus problems, catarrh and headaches, are suitable for self-treatment because of the power of this therapy.

Reflexology Treatment for Problems During Pregnancy

After carrying out a general treatment, special attention should be given to the named reflexes for the following problems.

Problem	Reflex
Fatigue	Thyroid reflex; if there is fatigue, the best treatment is rest
Morning sickness	Pituitary, thyroid, adrenals, stomach and intestines
Swollen ankles	Endocrine glands, bladder, ureter tube and kidneys
Constipation	Small and large intestine (paying special attention to the sigmoid flexure and anus) and the solar plexus
Flatulence	Stomach, small and large intestine
Insomnia	Brain, solar plexus and gentle massage to both hands

Osteopathy

Osteopathy is a system of medical therapy that uses the manipulation of the joints, the spine in particular, to treat disease. The system was devised in the United States by Dr Andrew Still, just over 100 years ago. He was a practicing doctor who had also trained as an engineer, and, as a result, developed an interest in the human body as a machine. He tried to figure out how defective parts of the body could hinder its proper functioning, in much the same way as one does with a machine with moving parts. He became convinced that good health depends on the proper alignment of the spine. The spine plays a vital role in supporting the whole structure of the body, linking its parts and carrying the spinal cord as well as providing the connection with the muscular systems. When any of the vertebrae get out of alignment, we fall ill.

Animals are instinctively aware of the importance of the spine. They take the time each day to stretch, arching the back and then making it concave, which allows the vertebrae to correct their alignment each time. Human beings are notoriously lazy about such things. All too often, we sit slumped in a chair, hunched over a desk or behind the driving wheel of a car. In this way we put a daily strain on our backs, rarely bothering to take the exercise we need to keep both spine and muscles in good, mobile working order.

That we should suffer backache and rheumatic pains if we do not look after our spines is perhaps not surprising. But Andrew Still went further than that; he believed that the spinal cord controls all the other systems in the body, because of its links with the nervous system. Many of the symptoms of dysfunction, such as skin conditions, digestive troubles and headaches, are, according to Still's argument, the result of spinal vertebrae being slightly misplaced. Still believed that if one found the disturbance and corrected it, good health would be restored.

Still was a doctor, and although at the time his argument seemed strange, people listened to him. It was not long before enough followers adopted his methods to establish the American School of Osteopathy in Missouri. The theory behind osteopathy was not, in fact, new. It is very ancient, going back as far as the ancient Greeks and Romans, both of whom set great store by a healthy body.

Although less popular than conventional physicians, doctors of osteopathy are actually licensed to prescribe drugs, perform surgery and do everything else that medical doctors do, as well as manipulate the spine and joints.

The manipulation of the joints, in order to keep the body mobile and healthy, can be especially beneficial during pregnancy when there is additional strain on the back, hips and knees due to the extra weight of the baby, and the softening effect on the joints by the hormones of pregnancy.

Osteopathy is most helpful for people with any kind of spinal problem such as low back or neck pain. These problems probably account for well over half of an osteopath's clients, many of whom will have been referred by their family doctor. Many other problems can be helped by osteopathy too. Tension headaches caused by contraction of the little muscles that lie at the base of the skull can be treated, and sports injuries also account for a large part of an osteopath's caseload. These may not necessarily be related directly to the spine but can concern joints of the feet, ankles, knees, hips, wrists, elbows or shoulders.

Osteopathy can have surprising results. It can even help cure problems of the internal organs which one would never have connected with the spine. Patients have reported success with treatment for indigestion, bronchitis, asthma and even circulatory disorders. A good osteopath can work wonders, producing results in a matter of minutes that several weeks of bed-rest might never achieve. This is one of the complementary medicines with the greatest degree of success, and undoubtedly has a positive future.

Its Role in Pregnancy

Many women suffer from backache in pregnancy. This is because high levels of progesterone have a softening effect on the tendons and ligaments of the body, allowing the joints to expand in order to make room for the growing baby and preparing the body for the rigors of labor. This has a particularly dramatic effect on the spine and the ligaments supporting the spine. The softening, together with the increasing weight of the growing baby, puts a tremendous strain on the spine which often causes backache. The typical posture adopted by a woman in advanced pregnancy is leaning backward, which adds further strain on the lower joints of the spine.

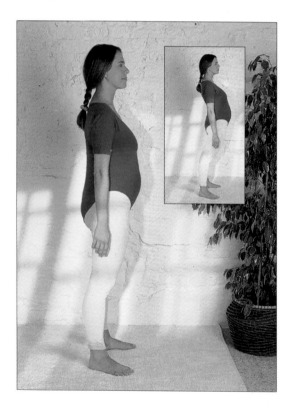

Above. *Keep tail tucked in when standing, walking or sitting. A hollow back (see inset) leads to backache.*

The Consultation

The first consultation with an osteopath starts with a medical history, followed by a detailed physical examination, noting the way in which you hold yourself when you stand, sit and lie, as well as the way in which you move. All this tells the trained osteopath a great deal about the state of your spine. The range and quality of your movement in certain joints will be examined, and the osteopath will then feel the soft tissues, muscles and ligaments to assess whether they are healthy or stressed.

This information may be enough for the osteopath to decide how to treat you. The osteopath may decide not to treat you if you are in need of surgery, or if there are symptoms of your disorder that are outside the sphere of osteopathy. You may be referred to another practitioner.

Some osteopaths also like patients to have an X-ray to confirm a diagnosis. This is not possible, however, if you are pregnant.

If examination shows that your condition is suitable for treatment by osteopathy, the osteopath will outline its course for you. The number of sessions required will obviously depend on how the osteopath sees the problem, but in general a chronic condition may well require several sessions whereas a recent and acute problem may be dealt with straight away.

An individual treatment lasts between twenty and thirty minutes. Osteopathic treatment is generally painless, though it can be uncomfortable if you are already in extreme pain, and you may feel worse after the first treatment. Some patients, however, find treatment both relaxing and enjoyable. There are several techniques that an osteopath may use (*see Osteopathy Treatments box opposite*). In addition to the treatment that you receive, the osteopath may also suggest ways you can help yourself including taking exercise to help ease a problem. Your habitual posture may exacerbate an existing condition, whereas adopting a better posture might ease it or even encourage it to be corrected. Your practitioner may also recommend relaxation. You may have difficulty in relaxing your joints and muscles, which is adding to their taut, stiff condition; in such instances the osteopath may teach you relaxation techniques that will help your particular problem.

Osteopathy Treatments	
Type of Treatment	What It Does
Massage of soft tissue	*Relaxes taut muscles and improves circulation*
Gentle repetitive movement of joints	*Increases the mobility of joint and reduces tension in surrounding muscles*
Correction of malfunctioning joint by guiding it rapidly through its normal range of movement	*Releases malfunctioning joint, producing clicking that many people associate with osteopathy, and corrects misalignment*

What You Can Do at Home

There are several things you can do at home or behind the wheel of a car to help ease a back problem. Do the following simple exercise regularly to ease the shoulders, which are prone to stiffness from stored tension. Shrug your shoulders toward your ears and then roll them backward, with the head slightly forward. Do this three or four times and you will feel the neck relaxing gently. Also try the exercise opposite daily to maintain mobility in the spine.

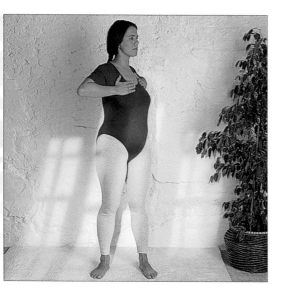

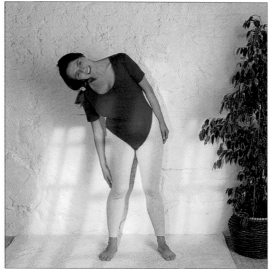

1 Fix the pelvis by keeping weight on both feet and swing shoulders alternately left to right, gently but as far as possible. This maintains mobility of lower joints and encourages good muscle tone and relaxed ligaments.

2 Without bending backward or forward, slide your hand right down the thigh; then reach three or four times. Repeat on other side. This stretches back muscles and ribcage, improving movement and breathing.

3 Push backward with the elbows, shoulders and head to feel a stretch between your shoulder blades (left). This increases mobility in the upper spine and neck.

4 With feet apart, droop from waist with neck, head and arms floppy, reaching as far as you can (below).

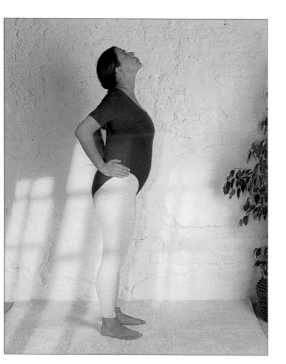

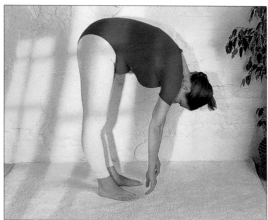

Craniosacral Therapy

Craniosacral therapy is a complex and subtle therapy which has evolved from straightforward osteopathy. Like osteopathy, you may find it particularly helpful during your pregnancy. In craniosacral therapy, the bones of the skull and upper neck are gently manipulated. In this way, the rhythmical pulse of the cerebro-spinal fluid is used as an aid to both diagnosis and treatment. This pulse is felt as very slight, rhythmical movements, first of expansion and then of contraction.

This system of treatment was developed by a conventional osteopath toward the end of the nineteenth century. William Sutherland was convinced that he could diagnose and treat all sorts of disorders simply by feeling his patients' skulls.

Although craniosacral therapy is gaining in popularity, there are few osteopaths nowadays who specialize in this branch of osteopathy alone. Many of them, however, use it as an extra variation in their treatment. It is generally used as part of the overall treatment and is so gentle that patients are hardly aware of what is being done to them—only of a gentle and pleasant massaging of their head.

Craniosacral therapy is particularly helpful for some treatable eye conditions, facial pain and persistent headaches, including migraines. Some cranial osteopaths have claimed good results in treating certain conditions that are usually thought to be resistant to treatment, such as epilepsy and deafness. Craniosacral therapy has also been useful in the treatment of autistic children and newborn babies; it has proved particularly successful with those babies who have experienced a difficult birth.

Chiropractic

Chiropractic is a manipulative therapy with similar origins to that of osteopathy. Using some of the same techniques as an osteopath, a chiropractor aims to correct disorders of the spine, joints and muscles by the manual manipulation of the patient's body. The main difference between the two is that a chiropractor relies more heavily on X-rays, than an osteopath, as well as using conventional diagnostic methods of blood and urine tests. Also chiropractors manipulate by thrust exerted on a joint, rather than by leverage. Basically, a chiropractor aims to do three things, including: correct bad posture, restore the function of the spinal and pelvic joints, and correct any interference with the nervous system that has been caused by deviations of the spinal and pelvic joints.

Most of a chiropractor's patients come for help because they are suffering from some sort of musculo-skeletal pain, particularly neck and lower back pain. People who have sustained whiplash—when the head is thrown back abruptly—as a result of a car accident are also commonly seen by chiropractors. Other ailments that are often treated by chiropractic include: headaches caused by the contraction of the neck muscles, strained muscles, sprained joints, damaged ligaments, tennis elbow, wrenched knees and damaged tendons.

Although a very old therapy, today's understanding of chiropractic is based on the work of a Canadian "magnetic healer" called Daniel David Palmer, who treated his office cleaner for deafness. The cleaner claimed that he had become deaf when he felt a click in his back while bending down. Palmer discovered that some of the small bones in the man's spine were out of place. He manipulated them and the cleaner's hearing was restored.

As a result of this Palmer studied the anatomical and physiological basis for such cures more deeply and developed a philosophy of treatment known as chiropractic. He went on to found the Palmer School of Chiropractic in Iowa.

Since Palmer's day, chiropractic has come in for a good deal of opposition from the orthodox medical profession. Only recently have many conventional doctors accepted that certain health problems can indeed, be caused by interference with nerve transmission brought on by deviations in the spine. In spite of this lukewarm reception by conventional medical practitioners, chiropractic has flourished, largely as a result of enthusiasm from its grateful patients. Nowadays, there are thousands of registered chiropractors and chiropractic is one of the most widely recognized complementary medical professions. The result is that more and more doctors are referring their patients to chiropractors for treatment of back pain.

Its Role in Pregnancy

Many women suffer from backache in pregnancy. According to chiropractors, this is caused by the increased weight of the baby on the spine and the pregnant woman's difficulty in maintaining her balance. Changes also occur in the pelvis and in the sacro-iliac joints (joints at the base of the spine)—both in pregnancy and in childbirth—which can cause back pain. Chiropractors can help ease this common problem for you.

The Consultation

At the first consultation, the chiropractor will take a detailed medical history, as well as details of the current problem, then will examine you thoroughly and will identify areas of pain, tenderness or muscle spasm. The therapist will probably want to take an X-ray in order to clarify the state of your spine, but you should decline this if you are pregnant or hope to be so (*see page 89*). As a result of all the information gleaned, the chiropractor will then decide whether you would be better off seeking conventional treatment for a particular disease or fracture, or whether chiropractic is the answer.

Treatment does not usually begin until after a full diagnosis has been made. It is conducted on a special chiropractic couch and involves various manipulative adjustments to the body. These should not be painful, and, in fact, you may feel immediate relief from pain. It is possible, however, that you may not feel any relief until after three or four treatments. In general, chronic cases need more treatment sessions than acute problems.

What You Can Do at Home

There is nothing you can do at home in the way of actual self-manipulation of joints. A chiropractor will often give advice, though, on other things that you can do to help the treatment, such as diet, exercise and rest. The therapist may also suggest other treatments, such as massage, posture training, heat treatments or yoga.

Alexander Technique

Alexander technique has been called a method of posture training which endeavors, through a series of very gentle exercises and movements, to correct posture, taking personal conditions into consideration. The aim is to re-educate the body so that it assumes new, healthier stances, ridding the body of the harmful posture habits which are thought to be stored in the unconscious memory.

Its founder, the actor F. Matthias Alexander, was born in Tasmania in 1869. He found himself habitually losing his voice on stage and discovered that he could cure the problem by improving his posture. This simple discovery became the starting point of an entire system of retraining the body's movements and positions, and today there are Alexander technique schools and training centers all over the world. Devotees claim that the technique can help improve health and can promote resistance to stress. Conditions for which success have been claimed include depression, anxiety, headaches, hypertension, respiratory problems, exhaustion, arthritis, back trouble and digestive disorders.

Its Role in Pregnancy

Pregnancy can cause you to adopt postures which may not be comfortable or conducive to a trouble-free pregnancy, particularly as your body undergoes such a complex set of changes. The Alexander technique will help you make minor adjustments to your posture and will make you more sensitive to your growing body's demands.

The Alexander technique will help you to adapt your ways of moving as you change shape, so that you are made more comfortable without endangering your baby. In particular, it will help you to use your body correctly so that backache—for so long assumed to be an inevitable part of pregnancy—may be entirely avoided.

And finally, it will help you prepare for the birth, thus making it as natural a process as possible. It teaches you to stay upright during labor and to move in a relaxed way by consciously releasing tension. Tension increases pain, which may result as an unthinking reaction to it. If you are relaxed, you can learn to cope with the pain and to allow the natural process of labor to proceed.

The Lesson

Practitioners of Alexander technique are called teachers, not therapists and the people they teach are called pupils, not patients. First of all, the teacher will watch how you use your body. Children move naturally, but most of us develop bad habits as we grow up; by adulthood, these bad habits become firmly ingrained. The teacher's aim is to show you how to change these bad habits and regain the ability to use your muscles with the minimum effort and the maximum efficiency. The teacher will retrain you to perform a whole range of everyday tasks—opening a door, getting in and out of a chair, getting in and out of the car, sitting at a desk, even answering the telephone.

All this is done by the teacher gently manipulating your body into more natural positions while you are standing, sitting or lying down. This is accompanied by verbal instruction that will help you become more aware of your own posture and will help the natural mechanisms of poise to function more freely. Gradually, as you practice better posture, you will be able to release inbuilt tensions and learn to use your body correctly. The teacher will use no force—just a series of gentle manipulations and subtle adjustments.

A lesson lasts about thirty to forty-five minutes. It is usual to have a course of thirty lessons, after which you should be able to continue on your own.

What You Can Do at Home

Bad postural habits are usually so ingrained that they feel entirely natural. As a result, it is virtually impossible, without help, to recognize what you are doing wrong. You may be able to see if your posture is slouched and awkward simply by watching yourself in the mirror, which is what Alexander himself did. Once you have completed a series of lessons with a qualified teacher, though, you will have learned enough to enable you to practice correct posture on your own.

Many Alexander teachers advise their students to relax for at least twenty minutes a day in the semi-supine position. This

position, which involves lying on your back on the floor with your knees bent and pointing to the ceiling and your hands resting on either side of the abdomen, gives the body complete rest and helps to relax over-tightened muscles. It is important to keep the neck in line with the spine, so you need to rest your head on two or three books. To get up, roll to one side, then raise yourself on to all fours and slowly stand up.

Below. *The habitual wrong way to sit at a desk (see inset) with head slumped forward, causing tension in back and arms, and shoulders unnecessarily raised. Tension in feet is transmitted to legs and the whole body is pulled out of natural alignment. Sitting poised (main picture) the neck is free of tension and head balances on top of spine, so back can lengthen and widen. You sit on sitting bones, feet supported by floor and any movement, forward or backward, pivots around hip-joints.*

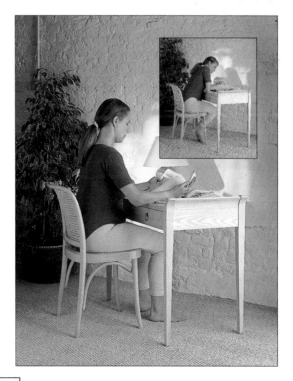

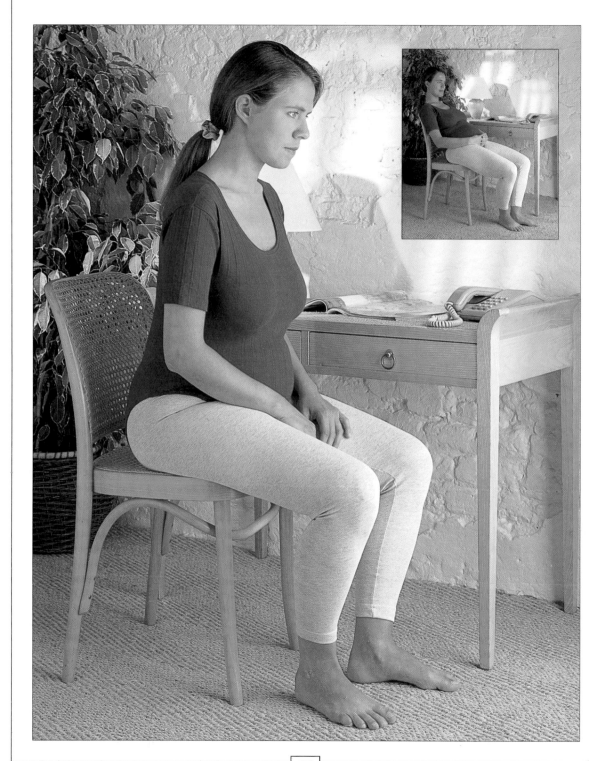

Left. *Slumped posture (see inset) causes backache. To prevent strain, sit on your sitting bones, allowing knees to go forward and slightly away from each other. Weight supported on chair: no need to tense feet and legs. Torso maintains length and width as you direct yourself upward, freeing neck and letting head go forward and up, to balance itself on top of spine.*

Right. *Getting up with your hands pushing down (see inset), head is pulled backward to compensate for unnecessary effort. When you consciously direct yourself to get up, let your neck be free to allow your head to go forward and up, leading the movement; body tilts forward, and weight easily transfers from chair to your feet.*

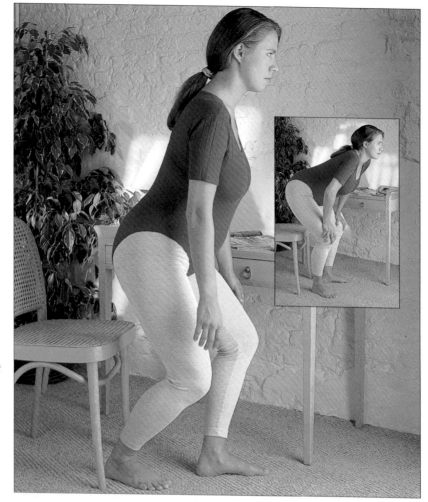

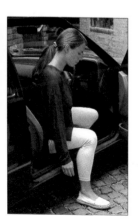

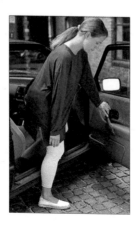

Far left. *To get into a car, stand facing forward at a slight angle to right. Leading with your head and letting torso tilt forward on hip-joints, lower yourself by bending legs. Transfer weight to right leg; lift left leg, placing it inside. Lower yourself further on to seat. Lift right leg and bring it in. Turn to face forward without twisting your spine.*

Left. *To get out, turn torso to right, pivoting on hip-joints. Bring right foot to floor. With head leading and back following, transfer weight onto this leg and get out without twisting your back or pulling yourself down.*

Yoga

Yoga is a Hindu philosophy which aims to achieve a state of physical and spiritual well-being through certain physical exercises and postures as well as through relaxation and contemplation. The word *yoga* is a Sanskrit word meaning, literally, "yoke" or "union," referring to the union between physical, mental and spiritual training that lies at the heart of yoga. This is a discipline that greatly benefits pregnant women. The *asanas*, or postures, which are practiced slowly with breathing and concentration, can prepare the body beautifully for the birth of a child, as well as creating a sense of peace and relaxation during the nine months of pregnancy.

Hatha yoga is the best known system of yoga in the West. It is designed to improve our physical health, balance and equilibrium. In India, yoga is a profoundly religious system of philosophy which has existed for thousands of years. In the West, many people take up yoga because it teaches relaxation, as well as increasing the body's flexibility and all-round fitness.

The postures that yoga teaches reduce stress, making you sleep better and leaving you calm, relaxed and with a clear, untroubled mind. In this way, yoga promotes both an inner and an outer harmony. The postures involve a slow, deliberate stretching and releasing of the muscles; each asana is done slowly and is held for a few minutes, allowing you to develop an awareness of your body and its internal and external tensions.

In the last few years, yoga has gained in popularity as a therapy in the management of a number of ailments, especially of stress and various stress-related problems. Yoga is recommended in particular for heart conditions and for asthma because it frees the chest and makes breathing easier. One of the reasons why yoga is so good for asthma sufferers is that correct breathing plays such an important part in its practice. According to the philosophy of yoga, breath embodies the individual's life force or *prana*. Although breathing is usually an unconscious action, it is possible to become aware of it and to control it. Most people tend to take short, shallow breaths, with little awareness. Yogic breathing encourages you to breathe more deeply and fully, filling the chest and the belly with each breath. The breath is let out slowly from the chest and then squeezed out from the belly. By becoming more conscious of the breath you can release tension throughout the body.

When you start, it is best to learn yoga from a qualified teacher and then you can practice at home. Yoga is most beneficial if it is done regularly—ideally, for just fifteen to twenty minutes every day.

Its Role in Pregnancy

It is important to tell your yoga teacher when you are pregnant, and equally important to inform your teacher if you have had any previous problems or miscarriages. It is not advisable to start yoga for the first time during your pregnancy without a teacher. Seek out a teacher who specializes in yoga for pregnancy. You should feel no discomfort or strain, and if you do, you should come out of the asana.

If you are already experienced in yoga, you should keep it up throughout your pregnancy. Your body secretes a hormone which makes your joints more flexible than usual, so you may notice an improvement in your asanas. Sitting poses are particularly good because they help to open up the pelvis before the birth. Standing poses are good too, because they strengthen the legs, which helps you carry the extra weight of the baby. It is important to listen to your body—only you can really judge what you are capable of doing and how best to adapt your asanas as you grow bigger.

Relaxation is important in pregnancy, and yoga is one of the best ways of training yourself consciously to relax. When you are properly relaxed, there are a number of changes that take place in your body. The heart rate decreases and because your heart is pumping blood at a slower rate, you will begin to feel your whole body slowing down. Your levels of both blood sugar and blood fat, which automatically increase in response to stress, will start to return to a healthy level. On the following pages are a number of positions which are of particular benefit to pregnant women.

Finding a Teacher

If you have individual yoga classes, the teacher will advise and supervise you, and will be able to design a routine to suit your individual case. But if you go to a class, tell your teacher that you are pregnant and then you will not be expected to do anything that might be difficult or dangerous. Some classes are intended specifically for beginners, others for more advanced students. Choose a class that suits you. If you are pregnant, it is important to let your teacher know, along with any relevant details about former problems or miscarriages. This is very important as there are some poses that you should not attempt.

There are yoga classes offered specifically for pregnant women; you might care to investigate this option, or perhaps seek out a teacher on an individual basis. Many classes are now organized by adult education centers, as well as by health centers and sports clubs.

What You Can Do at Home

Once you have been taught the basics of yoga by a qualified teacher, it is quite possible to practice at home. Many people prefer to keep on going to classes in order to make sure they are performing the positions properly and effectively. They then supplement the classes with additional regular practice at home.

Practice the postures on the following pages every day, if you can, to relieve tension and strengthen the muscles in your legs, pelvis and perineum in preparation for labor. Hold each pose, or continue alternating between poses, whichever is appropriate, for a few minutes or until it becomes uncomfortable. If you feel any pain whatsoever, stop immediately.

Squatting

Pregnant women should squat often—not only when they are doing these postures but at regular times throughout the day. Squatting strengthens the legs and the perineum in preparation for delivery. Becoming comfortable in this position may help you during labor because it is one of several effective positions in which to deliver a baby.

1 *Squat, with your knees apart and your heels on the floor, holding your knees in position with your arms (right). You may find this posture easier with your back against a wall. Stay in the squat until your legs feel warm. If at first your heels are not flat on the floor, support your buttocks on a folded blanket.*

2 *While you are in a squatting position, stretch the spine by pulling your head down gently (below).*

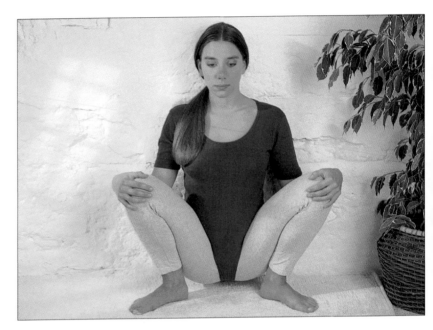

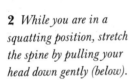

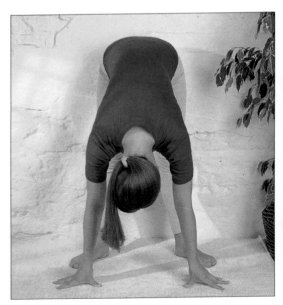

3 *To come out of this posture, slowly raise your buttocks and let your body hang from the hips (right). Hold this position for a moment, then stand up slowly, lifting your head first. Take a deep breath.*

Upper Thigh and Pelvic Stretch

This posture helps open the pelvis and strengthens the pelvic and thigh muscles that aid a comfortable delivery.

1 *Sit with both legs straight in front of you. Bend the knees out to the sides and draw the heels in toward the groin, joining the soles of the feet together (right). Then, holding the ankles, bring the feet as close to the perineum as is comfortable. Press the feet lightly together, keeping the knees level.*

2 *Place the palms on the floor behind the hips and stretch the back of the body upward (below). Hold for a few minutes then relax. Take a cleansing breath.*

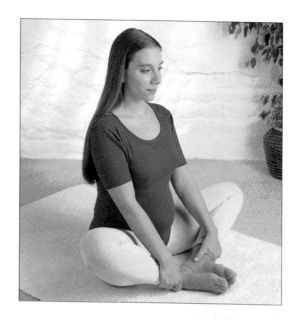

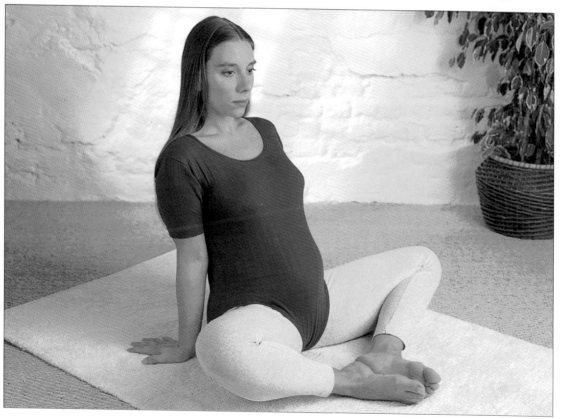

Standing

This involves alternating two poses—one in which you stand tensely and one in which you stand relaxed. They strengthen and tone the muscles and release tension.

Leg Lifts

This pose strengthens and tones the pelvic, abdominal and leg muscles. However, you may only feel comfortable doing this during your first trimester; after that, the pressure of the baby on the blood vessels against your spine will make lying on your back uncomfortable, so concentrate on this posture during the early months.

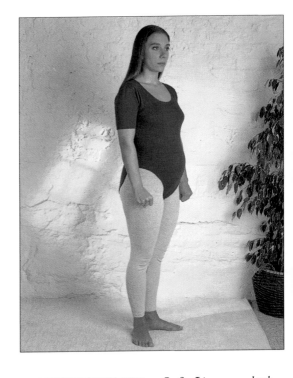

Right. *Stand with the pelvis tucked under, ankles together and feet at about 90 degrees. As you breathe in, tighten the legs, buttocks, arms and abdomen. Hold for a minute or two, breathing normally, then release.*

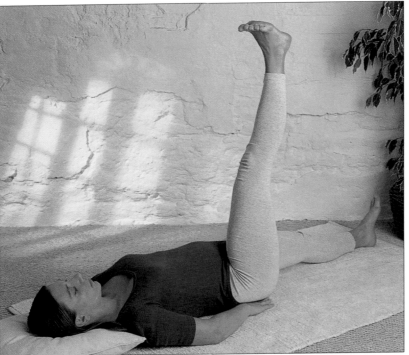

Left. *Lie on your back and breathe in. You can put a slim book or a small cushion under your head if you find this more comfortable. Then, using your hands to cushion your coccyx bone, breathe out and slowly raise one leg, only as far as is comfortable. Lower the leg as you breathe in. Raise the other leg as you breathe out. Continue in this way, raising and lowering each leg in turn as is comfortable.*

Cat Posture

This posture relieves the pressure of the fetus on the nerves and blood vessels of the lower pelvis and the upper thighs. It also relieves backache and improves spinal flexibility. The cat posture also helps to strengthen the spine.

Kneel squarely on all fours with your hands directly beneath your shoulders and your body and head parallel to the floor.

1 This kneeling position should provide a firm base. Take a breath in and as you do so slowly drop your back. Then spread your buttocks and raise your head and neck, keeping the face relaxed throughout.

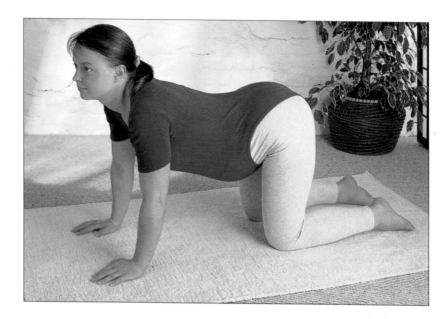

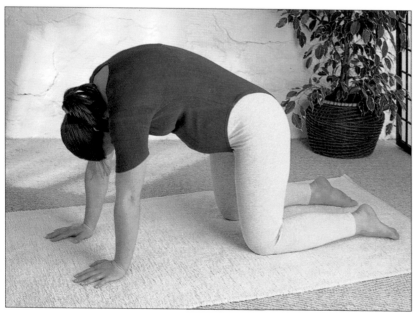

2 As you breathe out, tuck your pelvis under, arch the spine and lower your head. Repeat several times, alternating a concave spine with a curled-up one. Slowly build up to ten times, if that feels comfortable. This pose can be done right up until you go into labor.

Meditation

For centuries in India and in much of Asia, meditation has been practiced as a means of achieving spiritual enlightenment. It came to prominence in the West in the 1960s when many pop groups—most notably the Beatles—became interested in it as an alternative way of dealing with life's problems. But this ancient Eastern art can also be used to help alleviate the natural anxieties and stresses of pregnancy.

Meditation is a natural state of inner quiet developed through simple techniques such as watching the flow of your breath or by silently repeating a sound, such as *Om*. Long-term benefits of meditation include a greater equanimity and acceptance of life's ups and downs; a sense of inner peace; greater sensitivity to one's own and others' feelings and needs; and a more joyful and positive attitude to life.

There are several different schools of thought on meditation, each with a different view on the goal of meditation and how best to achieve it.

How to Meditate

You may decide to try meditation on your own, or you may prefer to do it as part of a group. Most people find it impossible to begin meditating on their own and will benefit from being taught the initial basic techniques. These may include adopting special postures, either lying down or sitting upright, and receiving a mantra—a sound or phrase suggested to you by your teacher that is then repeated over and over again. But once you have learned the basic techniques, meditation at home is very straightforward. A basic meditation technique is described below, which you can try at home.

It is best not to eat or drink for about half an hour before meditating. The room you use should be warm, dimly lit and quiet. Make sure you are not going to be disturbed for at least twenty minutes. Find a comfortable sitting posture where your back is straight—this may be in an upright chair, on the floor or on a bed with a cushion beneath you and your back against the wall, or just using a cushion on the floor and sitting cross-legged. Hands rest in your lap, or on your knees, eyes are closed. Take a deep breath and feel at ease.

Begin to focus on your breathing, watching the breath as it enters and leaves your body. Watch the flow of your belly as it rises and falls with each breath. Your breathing should be entirely natural.

Now begin to count silently at the end of each out-breath. You breathe in, breathe out, count one; breathe in, breathe out, count two; breathe in, breathe out, count three, and so on up to ten and then start at one again. If you lose count or get distracted just start at one again. When thoughts arise, simply observe them and label them "thinking" and go back to your counting. Try not to get involved in your thinking, just let the thoughts be like clouds passing in the sky. Make sure your back is straight but relaxed and you are at ease. You cannot meditate if you are feeling tense.

After five minutes, change the counting so that you are silenting counting at the beginning of each in-breath. You count one, breathe in, breathe out; count two, breathe in, breathe out; count three, breathe in, breathe out, and continue up to ten and then back to one again. This deepens your concentration and awareness of breathing.

After a further five or ten minutes you can drop the counting and just watch your breath, being at one with the flow. As you do this, become aware of the rhythm of your breath in common with the rhythm of the universe—each of the seasons, the tides, the breath in each being.

When you are ready, become aware of the cushion beneath you and the room you are in and the world outside the room. Gently open your eyes and have a good stretch. You may find it difficult to concentrate at first, but it will become easier with practice. Just meditate for as long as you can to begin with.

Relaxation Techniques

Like meditation, relaxation relieves stress and tension. Deep relaxation has a number of beneficial physical side-effects including helping to lower blood pressure; stress-related hormones such as adrenalin, are calmed and eased; the metabolism slows down; the sympathetic nervous system activity is decreased while the parasympathetic system is increased. The muscles relax. As the mind quietens and relaxes, fears, worries and the sense of being overwhelmed decrease. In their place, the ability to concentrate increases, as does efficiency and clear-headedness. Emotionally we feel more stable and whole, less needy or demanding. Anger is decreased, as is possessiveness or rejection.

With long-term practice, the benefits of relaxation may also include better circulation, relief from frequent headaches, easier breathing and a cure for insomnia. It offers a better alternative to tranquillizers, sleep-ing pills and antidepressants.

There are a number of straightforward relaxation techniques which can be learned and it is advisable to seek the help of an instructor initially. Outlined below is a simple relaxation technique that you can try at home. This can be read on to a cassette tape or have a friend read it to you. You may like to play some quiet and gentle music in the background.

Make sure the room you are using is warm, dimly lit and quiet, and that you will not be interrupted for at least twenty minutes. Have a blanket to lie on, a small pillow for your head and a light blanket to cover you. Lie down, arms by your sides, with the palms facing upward and feet slightly apart. During the later months of pregnancy you can lie on your side, with the top leg bent and a cushion under the knee. Release any restrictive clothing, remove your watch, jewellery, glasses or contact lenses; close your eyes and take a deep breath.

Begin by becoming aware of the rhythm of your breath as it enters and leaves your body. Then begin to relax each part of your body, starting with the right foot, breathing into any tension and releasing it. Work up your right leg, then the left foot and leg. Then relax your buttocks and pelvis, and work up each part of your back. Breathe into and relax your abdomen and chest. Starting with the right hand, relax your arm and shoulder, then your left hand, arm and shoulder. Breathe into and relax your neck, then each part of your face and the whole of the back of your head. Take a deep breath.

Feel your whole body as totally relaxed and heavy. Return to watching the natural flow of your breath, becoming absorbed in the rise and fall of your body as the breath enters and leaves.

When you are ready, begin to move your fingers and toes, take a deep breath and a good stretch. Come up slowly.

Their Roles in Pregnancy

Anything that allows you to relax will be of benefit during your pregnancy and both meditation and relaxation certainly achieve this. Exciting as it is, pregnancy is a stressful time for many women and their partners, and the value of both practices is that they are solvents of stress. As the mind is made to relax, so the body calms down too, which is good for both mother and baby.

What You Can Do at Home

Once you have learned how to meditate you will be able to practice on your own. You may find it helpful to play suitable music. Special meditation and relaxation tapes are available from specialist book shops and from some health food stores. As you become better at it, you will probably find that you can slip into a meditative or relaxed state virtually anywhere—not just at home but also on the bus, on the train, between household chores or even in your lunch break.

Visualization

Creating mental pictures to cure disease and to alleviate anxiety is a technique that has been used in many parts of the world for a great many years. It has tremendous potential for you and your unborn baby.

In visualization therapy, a patient is encouraged to draw a picture in their mind that will act as a stimulus for positive feelings about self-image, health and future life. It is felt that this will, in turn, be of enormous benefit to the individual's health and will speed up the natural healing processes.

Visualization therapy is not new. It has been used by witch-doctors in Africa and South America from early times and also formed an important part of early oriental therapies. Visualization was practiced in ancient Greece, where it was considered to be a crucial factor in healing illness.

More recently, a good deal of research was done on visualization therapy, most notably with cancer patients in the 1970s by Carl Simonton, a doctor who practiced radiotherapy in Texas. He found that through visualization—creating images of an army of white knights on horseback fighting off the invading cancer cells, for instance—his patients were getting better. Each patient found images that worked for them—some would see a battle between the good forces and the invading forces, others would imagine the cells quietly leaving, or perhaps being lovingly dissolved in the bloodstream. They became quite convinced that patients who took part in this program lived about twice as long as those who did not, and that, in some cases, the progress of the illness was completely arrested.

Another American, Dr Bernard Siegel, who works as a surgeon at Yale–New Haven Hospital and teaches at Yale University Medical School, has done a great deal of work on visual images created by patients, both in dreams and in paintings. Dr Siegel believes that many people have the ability to heal themselves, if only they have the will to live and are prepared to take on the responsibility for their own health.

Many therapists believe that visualization can be used for many problems. As well as cancer, it has been used with some measure of success to treat asthma, heart conditions and phobias, and is thought to be particularly effective in pain relief.

There can be a positive effect from imagining the body healthy and well, or by visualizing the energy in the body bringing healing and comfort to painful areas. It can also be used during relaxation to generate feelings of calmness and serenity by, for instance, visualizing oneself in a very peaceful and beautiful place.

Its Role in Pregnancy

Visualization can be a useful tool in the relaxation and breathing exercises which are undertaken as preparation for labor. Apart from that, it can also be valuable to visualize yourself having an easy, trouble-free labor. You can visualize yourself going through the birth and having an easy, supportive and loving experience. Visualize your body relaxed and opening easily to allow the baby to be born. Visualize holding a healthy and happy baby in your arms. By doing this you might find you can release any fears or doubts you may have about giving birth. Some practitioners are convinced that if a woman believes she will have an easy labor, then she is more likely to experience labor in this way.

The Consultation

The therapist will ask for a detailed description of your problem, then you will be asked to relax in a comfortable position, either sitting or lying down.

When you are completely relaxed, the therapist will ask you to imagine a scene that in some way relates to your particular situation or problem. It may be a real scene which you remember from a painting, a film or a photograph, or it may be an imaginary scene, which is entirely the product of your imagination. As you describe the scene you are visualizing, the therapist will encourage you to describe what you are feeling. The therapist may then ask you to alter or change your visualization if it seems that a revised image will ease your particular problem.

What You Can Do at Home

In general, it is best to be taught the technique of visualization from a practitioner before going on to practice it at home. You might, however, try this simple practice at home. If the following imagery does not feel peaceful to you, then visualize yourself going to a place that is special to you where you feel soothed, loved and relaxed.

Find a quiet place to relax. Perhaps quietly play some soothing and gentle music. Lie or sit in a posture that is comfortable to relax in. Start by just watching the natural flow of your breath coming in and out of your body, until you feel relaxed. Now begin to visualize that you are walking along a beach. The sand is soft and golden, the water is very blue, warm and gently lapping at your feet. Palm trees fringe the beach. You are quite alone and you feel very peaceful and serene.

You lie on the beach at the water's edge, letting the water gently wash over you. With each wave you feel you are being cleansed and released of all tensions. All your fears and worries are being washed away and you are left refreshed and invigorated. You feel the baby inside you resting peacefully.

After a while you stand up and begin to walk down the beach. With each step you feel yourself getting stronger and happier. You feel the baby inside you and now you feel joy at the thought that soon it will be the two of you walking together along the beach. Let the image fade and become aware of the room around you. Take a deep breath and gently begin to move.

Hypnotherapy

Hypnosis is an altered state of consciousness, somewhere between wakefulness and sleep, when the conscious and subconscious minds are susceptible to suggestions. A hypnotherapist uses the patient's altered state of consciousness to activate the patient's own will, giving it increased power over mind and body. This increased will can have a number of positive effects including healing illness, causing the patient to relax, and preventing or alleviating pain.

Pain relief was, in fact, one of the earliest uses of hypnosis. As early as the 1820s, the public was familiar with the power of hypnotism to relieve pain, though many doctors remained sceptical. During the mid- to late nineteenth century, some surgeons took to using it for some operations. James Esdaile, a surgeon practicing in Calcutta, performed many operations with no anesthetic other than the use of hypnosis.

By the end of the nineteenth century, in spite of its obvious success, the practice of hypnotherapy declined, largely as a result of the arrival of quick and easy anesthetics, such as ether and chloroform. It is only in the last fifty years or so that hypnotherapy has been revived as a method of pain relief. Hypnotherapy has been used successfully in the treatment of headaches, some digestive problems, skin disorders, asthma, insomnia, phobias and many other conditions related to stress and anxiety. Hypnosis can also be used to treat a number of addictions, which include smoking, drugs and alcohol. Some conventional doctors, however, remain sceptical about the ability of hypnotherapy to cure disease, but even they do not usually dispute its use in relieving pain, particularly in childbirth, and in easing the effects of anxiety and stress by promoting deep relaxation.

Its Role in Pregnancy

Hypnotherapy can induce deep relaxation which is generally beneficial in pregnancy. It can also be used to ease the pain of labor. Research has also shown that hypnotherapy can be very helpful in shortening the duration of labor.

A hypnotherapist can teach you the techniques of self-hypnosis which you need to know before delivery. You can then use self-hypnosis during labor to help you relax and to ease the pain. You might like your partner to be involved in this—both learning the techniques with you and helping and encouraging you to put them into practice when the time comes.

The Consultation

At the first session, the therapist will take a detailed case history and will also discuss how you see your current problem. You will probably not be hypnotized at the first meeting, although the therapist may test to see whether you are susceptible. Most people are open to hypnosis but a few people are resistant.

At the next session, you will sit or lie down and the therapist will hypnotize you. This is usually done by talking to you calmly, slowly and quietly, and suggesting to you that your eyelids are beginning to feel heavy and that you are feeling sleepy. Sometimes the therapist will get you to focus your eyes on a particular object, which will increase your desire to shut your eyes. All this is actually quite pleasant and you will indeed feel rather as though you are dozing off.

While you are in this relaxed state, the therapist will ask you to think about the future in as positive a way as possible, perhaps suggesting that any worrying symptoms will soon clear up. Or you may be asked to take a look at problems from a new perspective. Sometimes the therapist can help to instil new resolve to deal with a particular problem , or pose well-chosen questions that will help you both to explore why illness has arisen in the first place.

Tell your therapist that you are pregnant and explain that you hope, perhaps, to be able to use the techniques of hypnotherapy for the relief of pain in the early stages of labor. Your therapist will tell you what he or she believes can and cannot be done. If you are one of those who are more susceptible to hypnosis than others, your therapist may well feel that your chances of effective pain relief during your labor are good.

A session usually lasts between thirty minutes and an hour. At the end of it, the therapist will either talk or count you out of the trance. You need not fear that you will be left in this state between sleep and wakefulness. The therapist would have absolutely nothing to gain from this.

What You Can Do at Home

A hypnotherapist will usually teach a patient to carry out self-hypnosis at home. This works particularly well if you are having trouble relaxing or if you suffer from insomnia and need regular, on-the-spot treatment to help ease this problem. It can also be extremely useful for pain relief in labor. Some therapists will provide their patients with a tape recording, which will provide the right trigger for going into a trance-like state.

Color Therapy

Color, like a number of therapies mentioned in this book, is a very ancient form of therapy. From prehistoric times to more recent ancient history, there is much evidence that man has made great and imaginative use of color as a treatment. Archaeologists have discovered that the Egyptians had special rooms built into their temples which were used for color healing. And in India, color continues to be used in gem therapy and Ayurvedic medicine.

At the beginning of the nineteenth century, the discovery of new drugs and advances in surgical procedure superseded the use of color, making it lie dormant for a time. It was revived through the work of S. Pancoast and Edwin D. Babbitt, and following their work, other contributors, through research, have reinstated color as one of the complementary therapies.

We are all profoundly affected by color. Color therapists believe that color not only affects our moods and feelings, but also affects the physical health and well-being of our bodies. The body, according to color therapy principles, absorbs color in the form of electromagnetic components of light, and then gives out its own aura of electromagnetism as a pattern of vibrations which can be discerned by a skilled color therapist. A healthy body gives out a balanced pattern of vibrations, while an unhealthy body gives out an unbalanced one. The aim of the color therapist is to administer the color or colors that the sick person lacks, in order to restore the color balance to this pattern of vibrations or aura, as it is sometimes called. Specific ailments can be cured by determining which colors you should be exposed to and which you should not.

The most important function within the human body, at all its various levels, is the transference of life energy or *prana*. This is absorbed into the body in many ways, including through the breath and through the food we eat. Prana vitalizes the etheric layer of the aura which surrounds and interpenetrates with the physical body.

The etheric is the blueprint for the physical body and contains the major and minor *chakras* and the *nadis*. The word *chakra* is from Sanskrit meaning "wheel or vortex of energy." Five of the major chakras are situated in line with the spine, the sixth with the brow and the seventh lies just above the crown of the head. Each of the major chakras contains the full spectrum of color with one color being dominant in each (*see page 82*). Apart from being associated with various parts of the physical body, each chakra is linked to one of the endocrine glands and this is the reason for their

The Chakras and Their Influences on the Body

Chakra	Where It Is Situated	Dominant Color	Parts of the Body Affected
Base chakra	At the end of the coccyx	Red	Legs, feet, bones, large intestine, spine, nervous system, gonads
Sacral chakra	Halfway between the pubis and the navel	Orange	Skin, reproductive organs, kidneys, bladder, circulatory system, lymphatic system, adrenals
Solar plexus chakra	Between the twelfth thoracic and the first lumbar vertebrae	Yellow	Pancreas (only the islets of Langerhans)
Heart chakra	Between the fourth and fifth thoracic vertebrae	Green	Heart, circulatory system, lungs, respiratory system, immune system, arms, hands, thymus
Throat chakra	The back of the throat	Violet blue	Nervous system, female reproductive organs, vocal cords, ears, thyroid and parathyroid
Brow chakra	At the center of the brow	Indigo	Eyes, nose, ears, brain, pituitary gland
Crown chakra	Just above the crown of the head	Violet	Pure consciousness, pineal gland, connected with mood and sleep

importance in treatment. The nadis are linked with our nervous system and are the fine energy channels through which prana flows. On a sunny day there is an abundance of prana in the atmosphere, hence the reason why we all feel so full of energy. On a grey dull winter day, prana is greatly reduced. When prana is in abundance, the nadis appear strong and upright, but when depleted they droop, rather like a plant that lacks water.

Prana is absorbed through the spleenic chakra. On entering this center, it is refracted into the colors of the spectrum which are then transferred to the appropriate major chakra. Color therapists will tackle any problem—mental, physical or emotional. They emphasize, though, that their approach is intended to be a complementary therapy in conjunction with expert medical treatment, not an alternative to it. Success has been claimed with such complaints as headaches, asthma, eczema, arthritis, insomnia, depression and stress.

Its Role in Pregnancy

There are various ways in which a pregnant woman can help herself. Your therapist will diagnose your problem and teach you what you can do at home, so that you can then continue the treatment yourself. The chart opposite provides just a few examples of how color can help. They rely heavily on the techniques described in visualization therapy (see pages 77–78). Please reread that section before trying any of the following.

The Consultation

During your first consultation a detailed case history will be taken including details of your lifestyle, diet and color preferences. An experienced therapist will be able to tune in to your electromagnetic field and detect any imbalance.

There are two ways in which color treatment can be given. The first is through the use of a color therapy instrument. From this instrument the treatment color and its complementary are beamed on to the patient's body through shaped apertures for a precise 19.75 minutes. There are contra-indications when using this instrument and it should not be used on pregnant women.

The second way in which color can be administered is through the technique of "scanning." The patient lies on a treatment couch and is put into relaxation. The patient's aura is then scanned by the therapist to feel for any energy blocks. When this has been completed, the therapist channels color through the hands into the patient, starting with the head and working down to the feet. This is the technique which is advisable to use during pregnancy.

What You Can Do at Home

Color can be absorbed into the body in a number of ways, some of which you can practice at home. It can be breathed in using visualization. Color can also be worn, in which case you should always wear white underneath, which acts as a filter and ensures that the color is absorbed into the body. The therapist may suggest what colors you should wear, as well as which color foods you should eat. And finally, you can visualize colors. Your therapist will teach you how to visualize those most appropriate for you to use while you are pregnant and during your labor.

Uses of Color Therapy in Pregnancy

Problem or Aim	Treatment Color	Recommended Method
Difficulty in conceiving	Red	Visualize red coming up from earth through feet and legs to base chakra, which is associated with gonads (ovaries in woman, testes in man), and back through ovaries and fallopian tubes to earth.
For peace and tranquillity	Blue	Imagine whole body bathed in beautiful blue light.
Tendency to miscarry	Orange	Breathe in orange to sacral center on inhalation, then visualize it going out through ovaries and back down legs to earth.
Insomnia	Blue	Visualize a beautiful deep blue, and, with each inhalation, take this color into your body. Imagine your body is a container which you are slowly filling with blue light. Try sleeping in a blue nightdress between blue sheets and have a low-wattage blue light burning during the night.
Depression	Orange	Breathe in orange. Do not do this late at night, as it is one of the energizing colors and might interfere with sleep.
To stimulate milk flow	Orange	Visualize sitting under an orange waterfall.

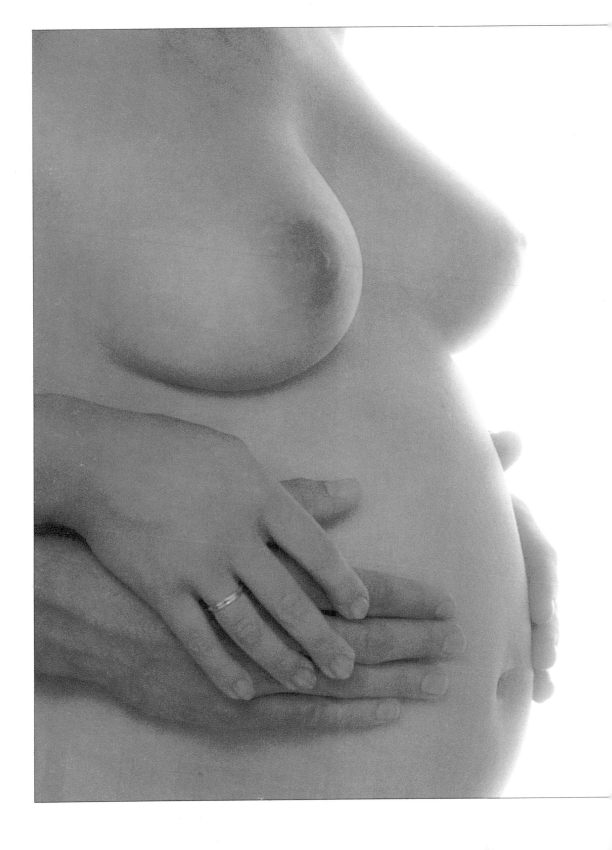

Part Two

The Pregnancy

～

art Two takes you through the three terms of pregnancy, the labor and birth, and the period immediately following delivery. Each chapter describes what is likely to be happening to you emotionally and physically throughout your pregnancy and outlines some of the complaints and conditions common to each trimester. Each chapter also explains how your baby is developing.

Many minor aches and pains can manifest themselves during pregnancy, and this Part shows you how each therapy can be used during each stage to provide relief, while helping you relax and reducing fatigue at the same time.

It is important not to exceed the stated dose for any of the treatments and to consult your therapist if you encounter any problems. Call your doctor without delay if you experience vaginal bleeding, severe abdominal pain, continuous and severe headache, possibly accompanied by blurred vision and swelling of hands and ankles. You should also seek medical attention if you experience excessive vomiting, in which it is impossible to keep down even water. Also be alert if your water breaks, or if you have a temperature of 38.5 degrees C (101 degrees F) or more. Sudden swelling of hands and feet and frequent urination accompanied by pain are also indications that you should see your doctor. Also see your doctor or midwife if you have felt no fetal movements for over twelve hours during the months when it is expected.

It is uncommon to experience very serious problems in pregnancy, but these danger signs indicate that something is wrong and should not be ignored. Most women will experience none of these and will progress smoothly through pregnancy and labor to the safe and happy birth of their baby.

CHAPTER ONE

Conception

❧

Conceiving a baby is a thrilling and momentous step in a woman's life and one which you and your partner will not have undertaken lightly. Undoubtedly, you will have given the prospect of having a child some careful thought beforehand and you will have discussed it with your partner. You will want to be quite sure that you are making the right decision—for you, your partner and your future baby. You will also want to do everything you can to help ensure both a fit pregnancy and a healthy baby.

If you are not already pregnant, then this is a good time to start pampering yourself to give you and your baby the best chance. Being fit and healthy before you become pregnant will ensure that you are prepared for the physical and emotional roller-coaster you are about to embark upon. Think about treating yourself to aromatherapy massage or an excursion to a color therapist. There may be no perfect time in your life to have a baby, but forethought gives you the chance to prepare for this major event before you conceive.

Preconceptual Care

Y ou need to pay close attention to your general state of health, your diet and your lifestyle before you decide to have a baby. The benefits of this care include increasing your chances of conception, maximizing your baby's chances of being healthy as well as giving yourself the best chance of having an easy pregnancy. Every pregnant woman worries about her own and her baby's health. Prepare for pregnancy, and you will have less reason to fret, which will make for a more relaxed pregnancy.

Diet

Your baby is totally reliant on you for its nutrition and you will no doubt adopt good eating habits as early as you can. These are habits that you should establish before you conceive. The benefits of healthy nutrition go without saying, whatever your age, whatever your circumstances, and whether you

are planning a baby or not. If you are thinking of getting pregnant, remember that you will soon have two people to consider, not just the one. Now is the time to increase your intake of fresh fruit and vegetables, fish, especially oily fish, complex carbohydrates, vitamins and minerals and herbal drinks. *Diet* in Part One outlines how you should eat throughout your pregnancy (*see pages 12–18*). Try to cut down on processed and junk foods, sugar, coffee and alcohol.

Now is the time to try to get your weight as near to the ideal level as possible. Once you are pregnant, it is not advisable to diet. Remember, too, that there are certain vitamins and minerals that are believed to increase the chances of conception for both men and women. Vitamin B6 for women and vitamin C for men are both thought to be helpful, whereas both sexes benefit from vitamin E and zinc.

Vitamins and Minerals Helpful to Conception

Vitamin/Mineral	Food Sources
Vitamin B6 *For women*	Organ meats, meat, fish, brewer's yeast, whole grains, wheat germ, vegetabl bananas, molasses, eggs, dairy products
Vitamin C *For men*	Fresh fruits, particularly citrus fruits and strawberries, all fresh vegetables, p icularly potatoes, green peppers and tomatoes
Vitamin E *For both sexes*	Most foods, particularly wheat germ, vegetable oils, fish, green leafy vegetables, whole grains and legumes
Vitamin A *For both sexes*	Oily fish, fish liver oils, milk, margarine, butter, eggs, organ meats, green and yellow vegetables, carrots, eggs, oranges, apricots
Zinc *For both sexes*	Oily fish, wheat germ, brewer's yeast, oysters, meat, walnuts, eggs, pumpkin seeds, molasses, onions, nuts, peas, beans

Exercise

If you lead a fairly sedentary life, you should try to take up some kind of exercise. This will not only ensure that you are as fit as possible before you become pregnant, but it is also important to get into good habits now so that you can keep them up when you are pregnant. Being physically fit will also be of some benefit in labor. Swimming is undoubtedly one of the best forms of exercise you can do when you are pregnant.

Sports to Avoid

If you are not used to exercise, do not embark on anything strenuous without having a word first with your doctor. There are some sports you should avoid during pregnancy, particularly any sport or exercise which involves sudden awkward movements or risk of falling such as riding, water skiing, skiing, windsurfing, climbing or scuba diving. Undertaking something entirely new is not a great idea and remember, it will be much easier to stay fit during your pregnancy if you are already fit before you became pregnant.

Drugs

On the whole, prescription drugs should be avoided during pregnancy, so if you think you might be pregnant, mention this to your doctor if drugs are prescribed for you. Remind the doctor every time you accept a prescription, and also check with the pharmacist. Some drugs can cause miscarriage, while antibiotics such as tetracycline can cause a baby's teeth to become yellow.

Even over-the-counter drugs are best avoided in pregnancy. Aspirin and some cough syrups, for example, contain substances that can be harmful to the growing baby. Obviously drugs can affect the fetus from the very earliest stages, so it is never too soon to start being careful. All illegal drugs, including cannabis, adversely affect your unborn baby, so should be avoided.

Alcohol

Alcohol can be highly damaging to the developing fetus. Give it up before you decide to become pregnant so that it will not be a source of worry to you.

Like drugs, alcohol can reach the fetus's bloodstream and is most harmful to the fetus during the first trimester, when all the vital organs are being formed. A baby born to a mother who drinks heavily may be afflicted with fetal alcohol syndrome. This entails a pattern of physical and mental defects including serious growth deficiency, malformed facial features, small heads, heart defects, abnormalities of co-ordination and movement and mental disability.

Smoking

Smoking, particularly in the first few months of your baby's life, is potentially the most harmful thing you can do to your child's health. Smoking is also strongly associated with infertility in women. You should therefore try to give up smoking before you get pregnant since it may take some time to kick the habit. There are other risks attached to smoking, including:

- increased risk of miscarriage, stillbirths and premature deliveries
- increased risk of congenital malformation such as cleft palate, hare lip and disorders of the central nervous system
- increased risk by nearly one-third of the baby dying in its first week of life if the mother smoked beyond the fourth month of pregnancy

- increased risk of a low birthweight baby because of the reduced amount of oxygen and the high amount of carbon monoxide in the baby's blood
- risk of crib death, or sudden infant death syndrome, doubles if the mother smokes during and after pregnancy
- increased risk of the child of a smoking mother suffering with infections of the respiratory tract, such as asthma, bronchitis and colds, sinus and ear infections
- increased risk of impaired ability to concentrate and learn, as well as impairing memory.

X-rays and Computer Terminals

If you are pregnant—or you do not know yet but you hope to be—you must inform any medical staff who plan to X-ray you. You must also tell an osteopath, chiropractor or dentist. Generally, you are strongly advised not to have X-rays during your pregnancy.

Human beings are extremely sensitive to X-rays, particularly in the first twelve weeks in the womb. The best advice to prospectively pregnant and pregnant women is therefore to avoid X-rays except in exceptional medical circumstances.

Few of us would disagree that new technology has brought a great change to most people's lives, particularly those of modern office workers. However, there is the question of whether computer screens or monitors give off enough radiation to harm a developing baby—medical opinion is still divided on this issue. Many can now be equipped with radiation screens and it would be advisable to use one, even if you are not planning to have a baby.

If you would rather err on the side of caution, avoid sitting in front of a screen if you are pregnant or you are trying to conceive.

Dental Care

During pregnancy you need to take good care of your teeth because much of your calcium supply is being diverted to meet the baby's needs. The high levels of progesterone produced by the mother in pregnancy tend to make the margins of the gums around the teeth softer and more spongy than usual, which predisposes them to infection. It is a good idea to visit your dentist at least once during your pregnancy and once while breastfeeding. Dental X-rays, however, should be avoided. If a dental X-ray becomes necessary, wear a leaded abdominal shield to protect the baby.

Genetic Counseling

There are certain medical conditions which may require genetic counseling. If you suffer from epilepsy, diabetes, asthma, heart disease or kidney disease, it might be a good idea to discuss your plans to get pregnant with your doctor and ask to be referred to a genetic counselor. No one will tell you not to have a child—they will simply tell you what the statistical risks are. You should also tell your doctor if you have a history of miscarriage, of fetal abnormality or of problems in previous pregnancies.

In addition, there are certain hereditary conditions which may lead you to worry that a child of yours could be affected. Many of these diseases can now be tested for at the preconceptual stage, to assess your child's chances of inheriting the disease. This sort of testing is known as DNA testing and can be done by a genetic counselor. Hereditary diseases that fall into this category include, among others, cystic fibrosis, Down's syndrome, Huntington's chorea, thalassemia, sickle cell disease, Tay Sachs disease and muscular dystrophy.

Health Checks

There are a number of routine health checks that are best done before you become pregnant. If any of the results are abnormal, then treatment is easier before pregnancy. A cervical smear, breast examination and a check for immunity to rubella are all a good idea.

If you are not immune to rubella, you can obtain a vaccination from your GP, then you should wait for at least three months before becoming pregnant.

You should have an HIV test during your pregnancy. There is a possibility that the HIV virus may be passed to the fetus, but there is medication available that can greatly reduce the transmission rate. Genital herpes is only a problem if the mother has an outbreak around her due date.

Age of Parents

There has been much interest recently in late motherhood, with more and more women postponing their childbearing until their late thirties and early forties.

From a simple biological point of view, the best time for a woman to have a baby is probably in her early to mid-twenties. However, biology is not the only consideration when it comes to having a baby, and women are tending to have their babies later for various reasons. Many women are not in stable relationships during those early years; the increasing efficiency and availability of contraception means that unwanted pregnancy can be avoided, and many wish to establish themselves in careers before becoming mothers. Being well-established in both career and partnership may serve as an advantage for older women who are embarking on a pregnancy at this stage of their lives.

Although it is undeniable that women become gradually less fertile as they get older, and that they run slightly greater risks of miscarriage and genetic defects, most older women have a healthy, if uneventful, pregnancy, a normal delivery and a healthy baby. The risks are reduced these days as prenatal care and screening improves.

Being older does, however, have undeniable advantages, including being more experienced, more mature, more patient and, hopefully, wiser. Being at least as old as your doctors and nurses can also give you an advantage when it comes to discussing your case and achieving the outcome you want.

Discontinuing Contraception

If the pill has been your method of contraception, you should have three normal menstrual cycles after stopping taking it before attempting to become pregnant. This will give your metabolic functions time to return to normal. There is no need to stop having sex in the intervening months; simply use some mechanical method of contraception, such as the condom or the diaphragm.

You are unlikely to become pregnant while taking the pill, but it is not impossible. If you suspect that you have become pregnant while taking it, you should see your doctor immediately, as there is a slight risk to the embryo from the hormones in the contraceptive pill.

If you become pregnant while you have an IUD *in utero*, it is usually advisable to have it removed as soon as possible if you wish the pregnancy to continue. If it is left in place, it can result in spontaneous miscarriage or premature delivery. Some doctors, however, elect to leave an IUD in place for fear of disturbing the embryo.

Therapies That Can Help Conception

Some of the complementary therapies are particularly relevant to women wishing to conceive. Men and women alike can benefit from the therapies' emphasis on relaxation, stress-relief and taking control of the process of pregnancy.

Relaxation

Some women experience difficulty conceiving because of tension and anxiety. Some, it would seem, have problems simply because they want too much to conceive, which produces a psychological block to conception. It is well known that signing the adoption papers can cause a woman, who had been having problems for years, to become pregnant as if by magic. Similarly, relaxation therapies—including massage, meditation, visualization and hypnotherapy—can all help establish the kind of atmosphere that is conducive to conception. Refer to *Meditation* and *Relaxation* in Part One for the techniques and information (*see pages 74–76*) that will help you and your partner at home.

Aromatherapy

There are a number of aromatherapy oils that can help promote conception. Those that are particularly relaxing are most useful. Keep in mind, however, that there are a number of essential oils that are contra-indicated during pregnancy including chamomile, rosemary and rose. They are fine to use until you are pregnant, but once you are, play it safe and avoid any on the proscribed list which you will find in *Aromatherapy* in Part One (*see pages 42–48*).

Aromatherapy for Conception

- *Luxuriate in a bath with aromatic oils of lemon balm, chamomile, rosemary, lavender or geranium—4 to 6 drops of essential oil well-dispersed in your bath. These will all aid relaxation before you go to bed.*
- *Essential oils of neroli and rose can be used as massage oils to help you relax and to regulate the balance of hormones. (Always dilute essential oils in a carrier oil before applying to the skin.)*
- *Essential oils of geranium and rose have a balancing effect on the reproductive system.*

Homeopathy

Ideally, both partners should have homeopathic treatment before conception to raise their levels of health, which will work to increase their chances of conception as well as preparing the mother for a healthy and trouble-free pregnancy.

As the mother-to-be, you will benefit from good "constitutional" treatment, which aims to treat your individual constitution rather than any specific condition or ailment. The individual's personality, emotional state and physical symptoms are all matched to those of the remedy. Each remedy has been proven on healthy people. This means the remedy has been given to a group of healthy people until mental and emotional symptoms occur. The homeopath then knows the range of that remedy and when this particular state is seen in a patient, the appropriate remedy, the constitutional remedy can be given—thus linking in with the person's immune system and raising their overall health.

Herbal Treatment

There are several herbs that aid fertility when taken regularly in an infusion. They can be helpful to both women and men, depending on what is causing the problem. Check *Herbalism* in Part One (*see pages 22–27*) to make sure that your herbal treatment does not include herbs harmful during pregnancy. You will also find information on preparing infusions. Note that Chinese angelica is suggested within the chart as helpful for enhancing fertility; it should be discontinued as soon as you become pregnant. If you do use other herbs from the proscribed list, stop once you are pregnant.

How Long Will It Take?

It is not uncommon to take a year to conceive, so do not worry if you do not become pregnant immediately. It is well known, in fact, that anxiety can impede conception. Meanwhile, make the most of whichever of the therapies appeals to you to reduce tension and to attain a state of tranquillity. Do ask your GP for a specialist referral if you have not conceived within a year of wishing to start a family.

Herbal Treatments to Aid Fertility

Hormonal Imbalance	Lowered Vitality	Tension and Anxiety
Vitex agnus castus	Ginseng	Cramp bark
(chaste tree or hemp tree)	Chinese angelica	Skullcap
False unicorn root	Cinnamon	Vervain
Chinese angelica	Ginger	Lemon balm
Wild yam	Winter cherry	Motherwort
Ginseng	Lady's mantle	Wild oats
Winter cherry	Lemon balm	Wild yam

Dosage: Take singly or in combination, a cupful of infusion three times daily

CHAPTER TWO

The First Three Months

✎

Your pregnancy has been confirmed and what you may already have known instinctively is now a fact, to be shared and celebrated with your partner. These early weeks are a very exciting time, especially if you are to be a mother for the first time. The first trimester of pregnancy, however, can be full of unknowns and uncertainties for both mother and father. Pregnancy is divided into three trimesters, each consisting of approximately thirteen weeks, with delivery usually taking place at around week forty. The first trimester covers the first thirteen weeks.

You may need reassurance and a good deal of emotional support, which is where complementary therapists can help—often more than the medical and nursing staff you will see as your pregnancy progresses. Quite apart from the therapies they offer, they are almost always willing to listen sympathetically, which is what many pregnant women need at this time. Relaxation and the relief of chronic fatigue and various aches and pains are all particularly responsive to the treatments offered by complementary therapists. Homeopathic remedies, delicious massages and a soothing cup of herbal tea often work wonders.

Your Body

There are women who claim that they can tell they are pregnant virtually from the moment of conception. They do not need to wait for any signs—they just "know." There are those who believe that this has something to do with the first secretion of the hormones of pregnancy. Not everyone can be so certain, however, and for most women, the outward signs are useful indicators.

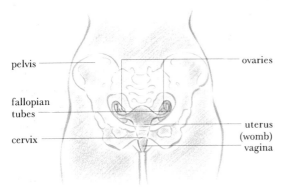

pelvis

fallopian tubes

cervix

ovaries

uterus (womb)

vagina

Above. *A woman's reproductive organs comprise the uterus, the fallopian tubes and the ovaries, the cervix and the vagina all contained within the pelvis.*

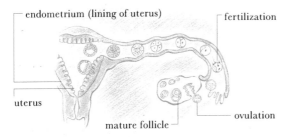

endometrium (lining of uterus)

fertilization

uterus

mature follicle

ovulation

Above. *This close-up of a fallopian tube and an ovary shows the development of the fertilized egg from mature follicle, ready to be released (ovulation), to its fertilization and implanting itself in the lining of the uterus. As it travels down the tube, the complexity of its structure increases all the time.*

Early Signs

One of the first signs of pregnancy may be nothing more than tiredness. Some women feel energetic, but most feel terribly tired in a way that they have never experienced before. You may find yourself so inexplicably tired, by mid-afternoon, that you just have to stop what you are doing and wait for this feeling of tremendous lethargy to pass. You may even find yourself dropping off to sleep, even though you got up only a few hours earlier. But, of course, tiredness can be symptomatic of a number of things.

Missed Period The first definite sign of pregnancy is a missed period, which is known as amenorrhea. While pregnancy is the most common cause of amenorrhea, it is not the only cause. You must not, therefore, assume that you are pregnant, though if you are trying to get pregnant it is probably the most likely reason.

Morning Sickness Many women suffer from morning sickness, which is caused partly by an increasing level of hormones circulating in the blood. The sudden rush of hormones can irritate the lining of the stomach, which manifests itself as nausea. Although it is called morning sickness and does indeed often happen in the morning, it can also happen at other times of day. Morning sickness can occur from about week six and rarely lasts for longer than the first sixteen weeks of the pregnancy.

Frequent Urination Another common early sign of pregnancy is an increased frequency of urination. A woman may notice this as early as one week after conception. It is caused by the swelling uterus pressing on the bladder, which lies very close to it.

Tender Breasts You may notice very early on a soreness and tingling of the nipples, together with a heavy tender feeling of the breasts. These may feel larger very early in pregnancy.

Taste You may also experience a characteristic taste in your mouth—often described as metallic—and your preferences for food and drinks may change quite markedly, sometimes even before you miss a period. Pregnant women often go off coffee, alcohol and fried foods, and may have strange new cravings—often cravings that they should resist because they are for sweet and high-calorie foods which may be low in nutritional value.

Testing for Pregnancy

You should wait until six weeks after your last period or two weeks after your period is due before taking a pregnancy test. This is because pregnancy tests taken too early can sometimes give false negative results and, rarely, false positive ones. You can buy an over-the-counter pregnancy testing kit and do it yourself or, if you prefer, you can arrange to have a pregnancy test done by your doctor, by a hospital or by a family planning clinic.

How Pregnancy Tests Work

Pregnancy tests work by detecting—and measuring—the amount of one of the pregnancy hormones, called *human chorionic gonadotrophin* (HCG), which is produced in the woman's bloodstream. The amount of HCG in a woman's body doubles every two or three days in the first six weeks of pregnancy. Manufacturers of the tests suggest that you use an early-morning urine sample because HCG is present in the bladder in its greatest concentration first thing in the morning.

Most tests work according to the principle of agglutination. The urine sample is mixed with an anti-HCG substance. If the woman is pregnant, the urine will contain HCG, which will neutralize the anti-HCG. The mixture is added to a suspension of particles coated with HCG. If she is pregnant, there will be no reaction because the anti-HCG has been neutralized, If, on the other hand, she is not pregnant, the particles are agglutinated (in other words, they clump together) by the unfixed (non-neutralized) anti-HCG. Some of the more recent tests are colorimetric tests, based on color changes. Done by a doctor or hospital, most pregnancy tests are generally fairly reliable.

Home pregnancy testing kits are also quite reliable, but you must follow the manufacturer's instructions carefully in order to obtain accurate results. Occasionally they fail to give accurate results for a variety of reasons including: doing the test wrong; doing it right but reading the result incorrectly; or doing it right and reading the result correctly, but the reagent substance fails to function properly.

A Negative Result

If the first test is negative, you should repeat the test a few days later, by which time the level of HCG (if you are pregnant) will have increased. If the second result is also negative, you are probably not pregnant. This can be a blow for a couple who are eager to have a child. It is important not to let a negative result cause any kind of rift between you. Most importantly, neither partner should blame the other in any way. Conceiving and having a baby is a shared enterprise and the ups and downs involved must be shared likewise.

Should this turn out to be more than a minor setback and should infertility prove to be a real problem, then both of you must talk to your doctor and make decisions jointly to see what can be done. Unless you have been trying for over a year, your doctor will advise you to go home and try again. This might well be the time to try some relaxing therapies, and try not to think and worry about conceiving, because this will be counterproductive. If you have been trying for a year, do not despair; it is common for many couples to fail to conceive in the first year. Anxiety itself can delay conception.

There is much that can be done nowadays and sometimes the obstacles to conception may be relatively minor.

A Positive Result

If the result is positive, you should make an appointment to see your doctor a couple of weeks later—bringing you to about eight weeks pregnant. These days you are not likely to be examined internally, but should you have an internal examination, the doctor will try to detect the softening of the genital organs and the increase in size of the uterus by using two fingers to feel the uterus while palpating your abdomen with the other hand. The test is generally 100 percent reliable after the eighth week, though if there is any doubt, an ultrasound scan a little later will resolve the question (*see page 99 for Ultrasound Scans*).

Diet and Exercise

Much of the advice given earlier on diet applies during this phase of pregnancy. Your nutritional intake has a profound effect on the health of your baby, so maintain good eating habits and keep in mind the old adage of eating for two, because you are! Therefore continue to eat plenty of fresh fruit and vegetables, complex carbohydrates such as whole grain bread, potatoes, rice and pasta as well as iron-rich foods such as leafy green vegetables, eggs, dried fruit, legumes and red meat. Keep up your intake of protein with dairy products, fish, lean meat, nuts or legumes, tofu and soy products. Drink mineral water and diluted fruit juices and if at all possible do not drink any alcohol. If you can manage it, do not smoke at all.

Before you embark on any exercise program in early pregnancy, check with your doctor that it is safe for you to do so. If you have a history of miscarriage or other complications, you should avoid exercise in the first three months. When you have the all-clear, though, you should take some form of regular exercise, preferably every day. This can be gentle and slow, but it should be regular. Exercise benefits both your mental and your physical well-being, helping you to relax and aiding circulation, which means that both you and the baby get plenty of oxygen. Being fit will also increase your chances of having an easy labor, as well as making it easier to, and more likely that you will, regain your pre-pregnancy shape after the birth of your baby.

Your Baby

Weeks three–four The blastocyst (a collection of cells in the shape of a sphere) implants itself in the lining of the womb.

Weeks four–five The blastocyst is now an embryo. It consists of three layers, from which all the body structures will develop.

Weeks five–six The embryo's head is forming. The heart is beating and the legs, no more than tiny buds at first, are growing.

Weeks six–eight All the internal organs are formed. Fetal length is 2.5cm (1in).

Weeks ten–eleven The baby is moving about a great deal, although you cannot feel it yet. Its eyes are formed and its fingers and toes are forming, but are still joined by webs of skin.

Weeks twelve–thirteen By now the baby's external genitals are formed. All its facial features are in place. Its muscles are getting stronger, which means that its movements are getting more vigorous. An ultrasound scan can pick up the baby's heartbeat, which is much faster than our own. Fetal length is 7.5cm (3in).

Your Feelings

The baby develops very quickly during the first three months of pregnancy, though there is little physical sign of this to the outside world. It may seem incredible to you that you are walking around with a tiny miracle developing inside you, yet no one else can tell. You may think you must look different—and yet you do not.

Even by the twelfth week you probably will not look any different to the outside world. However, you will be able to see all sorts of changes when you look at yourself naked in the mirror. Your nipples are probably bigger and the circles around them darker. Your breasts will be fuller and heavier. But put your clothes back on and no one will be any the wiser. Yet you will probably feel so different. Your breasts tingle. You have a sensation of fullness low in your abdomen. You want to urinate more often. You may feel slightly sick some of the time,

although some women do not feel sick at all. Pregnant women can run the full spectrum of emotions—of confusion, of joy, of wonderment, of anxiety—as they reflect upon their pregnancy; this is entirely normal.

Feeling Anxious

Nearly every parent-to-be—and most particularly the mother—experiences some anxieties about their impending role. Will the baby be all right? Will it be normal? Will the birth be OK? Will they be good parents? Will they be able to cope? All these worries are perfectly normal ones which many pregnant women and their partners seem to experience. They are not a sign of weakness or hopelessness, merely an indication that each of you is taking your prospective role seriously. Now is a time when each of you is reviewing your life and contemplating the new shape of the family unit.

What Sort of Childbirth?

Although it is a little early to think about what sort of childbirth you might prefer, it is a good idea to know what sorts of choices are available to you. Many prenatal clinics now provide their patients with birth plans for you to fill out and discuss with your midwife. Take some time to think about it, and remember that it is your body, your pregnancy and your baby; you are entitled to change your mind and no birth plan is fixed in stone.

For most normal pregnancies, there are different choices open to you for prenatal care and delivery of your baby. Most American women have their babies in hospital, while others are delivered by midwives in birthing centers or at home, usually by midwives. Home births are uncommon in the United States because of the fear that if a complication ensues, there may be inadequate time to get to a hospital.

Many hospitals have established "birthing rooms", outfitted to look cozy and home-like. However, births in a hospital almost always involve more technology than in a birthing center. Few women are deemed normal enough to qualify for the birthing room, and usually there is only one, so only one woman at a time can use it. Many women prefer midwives to obstetricians because midwives are trained to see birth as a healthy process rather than one fraught with complications.

Home Delivery If yours is a straightforward pregnancy, then home delivery may be an option you wish to explore. You will see the same midwife throughout your entire pregnancy and delivery, and you will be able to avoid medical intervention. Because you are in familiar circumstances, you may feel more relaxed and in control of the situation. And after the birth, breastfeeding will probably be easier at home than in a busy hospital room.

On the other hand, if you are at home it may be difficult to get help quickly if anything goes wrong. In addition, after the delivery, it may be more difficult for you to achieve the rest and peace that you will need, unless there is someone on hand to answer the doorbell and the telephone and to provide you with meals and drinks. If you already have children, they too will need looking after.

Hospital Delivery There are certain conditions which make hospital delivery necessary, including high blood pressure, diabetes, severe anemia and epilepsy. It is also necessary if any previous deliveries have included stillbirth, placental insufficiency, difficult forceps delivery and retained placenta. Other reasons include if your baby is breech or if you are carrying twins, if you are over 35 years old or if you are a rhesus negative mother, if you have had a cesarean section, or if you have placenta previa (placenta lying in the lower part of the uterus). Under these circumstances, you will probably feel more confident about the outcome of your pregnancy if you opt for a hospital delivery.

Hospital delivery does have its drawbacks though, including medical intervention you may not be happy with; you may feel intimidated by the medical staff and you may find hospital routine very disruptive and exhausting. However, some women enjoy the company of other new mothers at this time and they also relish the opportunity of doing relatively little for a short time at least.

Your First Visit to the Prenatal Clinic

At around twelve weeks you will visit your prenatal clinic for the first of many times. The main reason for your first visit is to ascertain whether your pregnancy and delivery are likely to be normal, and to run a number of routine tests to check on your general health. These will include weight, blood pressure, urine and blood.

You should also discuss any screening procedures that are considered advisable, such as ultrasound scans and prenatal diagnostic tests such as chorionic villus sampling, the triple alphafetoprotein (AFP) test and amniocentesis. You may be offered an ultrasound scan, which is usually done during weeks twelve to fourteen and is performed on an increasingly routine basis.

Ultrasound Scans

Ultrasound gives a photographic picture of the baby in the womb. The picture is made up of the echoes of sound waves bouncing off different parts of the body, and unlike X-rays, gives a detailed picture of soft tissue. An ultrasound scan is quick—it takes about five or ten minutes—and is completely painless. You will be asked not to pass urine beforehand and to drink lots of fluids so that your bladder is full and visible to the technician.

Oil or gel is poured on to your stomach and a special transducer (a hand-held scanner) is passed over the entire stomach area. This sends back signals, which can be seen on a black-and-white monitor. You will be able to watch your baby on the monitor as the technician scans over your tummy with the transducer. Seeing a picture of your baby in this way for the very first time is very exciting and somehow makes the fact that there is a person growing inside you very real. You may not be able to work out exactly what all the shapes mean, but the technician can point out the baby's head, limbs and organs to you. If the ultrasound is done after sixteen weeks, it may be possible to tell whether your baby is a boy or a girl. Be sure to tell the technician whether you want to know the sex of the baby or not; some parents want to know in advance, while others want to be surprised on the baby's birthday.

Scans are able to confirm a pregnancy from a very early stage; even before the first period is missed it is possible to pick up the fluid-filled sac implanted in the uterine wall. As early as six weeks after a missed period, it is possible to detect the baby's heart beating and three weeks after that, the placenta can be seen by ultrascan as well.

Why Ultrasound is Done

- *Determines the age of the fetus to within a week*
- *Measures growth*
- *Shows the baby's heart beating*
- *Shows any visible abnormalities of the baby, such as certain kidney or brain conditions*
- *Shows if you are carrying twins (or more) and if you will therefore need special prenatal care*
- *Locates the exact position of baby and placenta before having chorionic villus sampling or an amniocentesis*

An ultrasound scan is particularly useful if you have experienced any bleeding early on in your pregnancy and are worried about miscarriage. A scan indicating that the baby's heart is still beating will strongly reassure you of the successful outcome of your pregnancy.

Some research questions the validity of multiple scans. It has been suggested that multiple scans be limited to women at risk and that for the rest of us they be done only at strategic times.

Chorionic Villus Sampling

One test that you may be offered at this stage is chorionic villus sampling which can detect defects such as Down's syndrome and inherited disorders such as hemophilia, muscular dystrophy, cystic fibrosis, sickle cell disease and thalassemia. It cannot detect spina bifida.

The technique, which is done between weeks ten and twelve, takes about fifteen minutes. A narrow tube is passed into the uterus, through the vagina, to the outer sac surrounding the baby, known as the chorion. A small sample of the floating tendrils of the chorion, called the villi, is sucked into the tube, then taken away to be cultured and analyzed for information about

the baby's genes. Chorionic villus sampling is an earlier alternative to amniocentesis (*see pages 110–111*). The fact that it is performed earlier in the pregnancy, and that the mother therefore has the opportunity of an early termination of pregnancy in the event of a serious disorder being found, is probably its greatest advantage. Its disadvantages are that it is less accurate than amniocentesis and it is more likely to cause miscarriage.

Like amniocentesis, the test can identify conclusively the child's sex, which makes it an important test in cases where the risk of passing on gender-linked diseases is high. Needless to say, doctors are not willing to perform the test merely to find out if the baby is a boy or a girl. However, you may be able to choose between this and amniocentesis, which has a somewhat lower rate of miscarriage.

You will also have the chance during this first visit to say what sort of delivery you want, which is why it is important for you to have decided on your preferences. If you meet with any disapproval of your choice—perhaps you want a home delivery and your doctor does not agree—do not allow yourself to be put off too easily. Listen to reason, of course, but if you are confident that your decision is the right one, stick with it. Do try to reach an agreement with your health care practitioner if you can. However, if you are unable to come to a consensus, you may need to switch practitioners in order to plan your birth in a way that feels most comfortable to you.

It is as well, too, to voice your preferences at this early stage on such matters as pain relief, how long you want to stay in hospital, if that is where you want to have your baby, how you feel about episiotomy

---

Chorionic Villus Sampling is Done if:

- *Obstetrician suspects some abnormality*
- *You have already had an abnormal child*
- *There is a family history of abnormality*
- *You are above a certain age, usually 35*
- *You are a carrier of some hereditary disorder, such as muscular dystrophy or hemophilia, where a male child will have a 50/50 chance of inheriting the disease.*

(see page 142), if you are prepared to be induced if your baby is overdue and so on. All these things should be taken down and put on your file. This is your pregnancy, your baby, and—to a large extent—you are in charge.

However, many prenatal clinics these days supply their patients with birth plans, so that you can state your wishes regarding delivery, pain relief and amount of time spent in hospital, and have these wishes recorded in your notes. You may or may not have access to your medical records, depending on what State you live in, so it is a good idea to keep some notes of your own and take them with you when you go to the hospital or birthing center.

If all that sounds as though the first three months of pregnancy are some sort of ordeal, fraught with problems and difficult decisions, be reassured that it is a thrilling time when many women feel radiantly healthy. Although it is a time of enormous upheaval and change within your body, the great majority of women do not experience any problems at all. Those that do occur are not really problems so much as minor discomforts which most women accept as only a slight inconvenience brought on by their pregnancy. These can often easily be dealt with by one of the many complementary therapies available.

Therapies for Common Complaints

The great majority of women have healthy, normal pregnancies. It is undeniable, however, that many women in pregnancy can suffer from a number of minor complaints, most of which are uncomfortable and inconvenient, rather than giving rise to any major problems or to any real cause for concern. Complementary therapies can help with a number of these complaints. Morning sickness, for instance, can be helped with acupressure, acupuncture, color therapy, herbal treatments, homeopathy, shiatsu and yoga. For a comprehensive list of common complaints and therapies for all stages of pregnancy, refer to the master table (*Complaints and Therapies on pages 153–156*).

To take best advantage of any of these complementary therapies, you should have professional treatment first, or at least professional guidance to enable you to treat yourself at home. Although there are several therapies which require treatment by a practitioner—acupuncture, for instance— there are a few therapies, however, that can be administered as self-help treatments. Before you embark, reread the relevant section in *Therapies* in Part One and pay particular attention to any cautions or contraindications outlined under your chosen therapy. Both herbalism and aromatherapy use substances that should be avoided during pregnancy and there are certain acupressure and shiatsu points that should not be stimulated in early pregnancy.

If you do not gain relief from your chosen therapy, you will need to consult an experienced therapist. Alternatively, you could consider turning to one of the other therapies, perhaps one you have not tried before.

Homeopathy

In addition to the use of Tissue Salts (*see pages 31–32*), there are several remedies that you can try for some of the most common problems associated with pregnancy, including constipation, cystitis and morning sickness.

Homeopathic remedies are also suggested as treatment for hemorrhaging. Hemorrhaging signals a threatened miscarriage and must obviously be taken very seriously indeed. Seek medical attention but take the appropriate homeopathic remedies in the meantime. You will probably be referred to the hospital for an ultrasound to check that you are still carrying a viable fetus. If you are, you will be sent home and told to take things easy until your pregnancy is well-established, but there are certain homeopathic remedies that may be prescribed by a practitioner which can increase your chances of holding on to your baby. If there is a fetal abnormality, then, unfortunately, homeopathic remedies will not succeed in stopping the miscarriage.

Herbal Treatment

Similarly, there are several herbal treatments that you can use to try to relieve some of the most common complaints that are likely to affect you in the first three months of pregnancy. Probably the easiest conditions to treat yourself include nausea and sickness, heartburn, fatigue, constipation, cystitis, insomnia, thrush and varicose veins. You can also use herbal remedies, both externally and internally, to help prevent stretch marks.

If you have a threatened miscarriage, seek medical help, but there are several things you can do to help ease the problem if the baby is still healthy and strong. These include sipping a decoction made from one or a combination of herbs including false unicorn root, wild yam, black haw, cramp bark, raspberry leaves and squaw vine every fifteen to sixty minutes.

Pregnancy does not confer immunity from many common minor illnesses such as colds and flu. Since you may not be able to avail yourself of the usual over-the-counter remedies, you might like to consider some herbal remedies. Echinacea tincture can be taken at the first signs of a cold. Take a half teaspoon of tincture in a little water every two hours. For general relief of symptoms, take a cupful of yarrow infusion three times daily.

There are a number of herbal infusions which may be helpful with flu as well. If you have a fever, try a cupful of catnip, chamomile or lime flower tea three times daily. For a sore throat, an infusion of chamomile, either as a tea with honey, or as a gargle three times daily, can be soothing. To stimulate the immune system if suffering from an infection, try a cupful of echinacea tea and garlic every two hours. For a useful tonic during your recovery, take three cups of vervain tea daily.

For a comprehensive list of herbal treatments for most minor complaints in pregnancy refer to the Herbal Remedies Chart (*see pages 25–27*) in the *Herbalism* section.

Yoga

There are a number of yoga poses that help considerably with some of the common discomforts of the first trimester of pregnancy (*see pages 103–104*). The right angle pose is particularly good for relieving backache, commonly experienced by many pregnant women, and the thunderbolt pose is excellent for constipation and morning sickness.

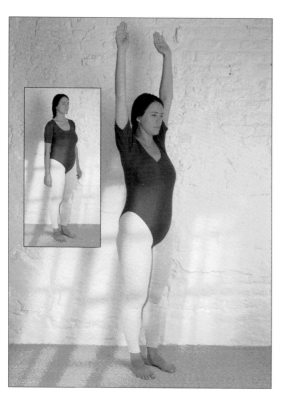

Backache

Right Angle Pose This pose is particularly good for backache. It rectifies poor posture and corrects curvature of the spine as well as being a wonderfully relaxing pose. As your stomach grows you might find it easier to do this pose with a chair in front of you, with the back of the chair nearest to you. You can then rest your hands lightly on the back of the chair for support when you bend at a right angle.

1 *Stand straight, with your feet together and your arms at your sides (see inset). Stand upright yet with your body relaxed.*

2 *Inhale as you raise your arms straight up, reaching up with fingers (main picture, left). Stretch upward, raising the trunk as well.*

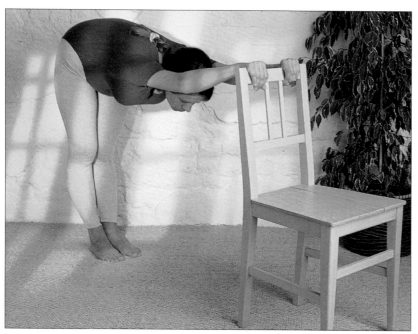

3 *Exhale as you bend your body at the base of the spine, so that it forms a right angle. Keep the spine and the neck straight. If using a chair, rest your hands lightly on the back (left). Breathe normally and remain in this pose for a few moments. Make sure your spine is straight.*

4 *Lift up gently, arms first. Come back to a standing pose. Repeat only as often as it feels comfortable.*

Constipation and Morning Sickness

Thunderbolt Pose This pose increases the efficiency of the digestive system and is particularly useful in cases of constipation and morning sickness because it relaxes the intestines and anal muscles. Practice after meals to help prevent indigestion.

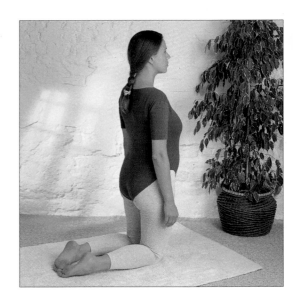

1 *Kneel up, with your feet behind and big toes crossed. Your knees should be together and heels apart (right).*

2 *Lower your buttocks to your feet, sitting between the heels (below). Place your hands, palm down, on your knees. Relax the abdominal muscles. Close your eyes, breathe gently and remain like this for a few minutes.*

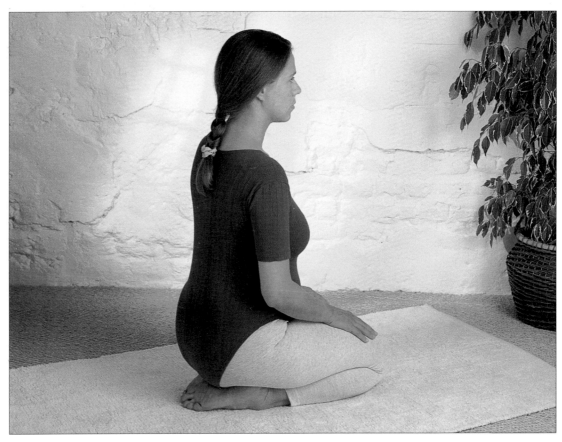

CHAPTER THREE

The Second Three Months

❧

During the second trimester of most pregnancies, from weeks fourteen to twenty-seven, many women seem to glow with good health and vitality. You, too, will most likely experience these sensations of well-being, when you feel full of life, literally, and you look as good as you feel. During this time your eyes will shine, your hair will be thick and lustrous and your skin will be clear.

By this stage of pregnancy, most women are no longer suffering from morning sickness and the overwhelming tiredness that seem to accompany those early weeks. You should have more energy, and in spite of your stomach, will be walking with a spring in your step. This is perhaps the most enjoyable phase of pregnancy; you are physically aware of being pregnant but the baby is not yet big enough to inhibit or change your movements and posture. And you have the benefit of hormones making your hair, skin and eyes shine with health. You will also perhaps be adjusting to the reality of sharing your life with another, very dependent person.

Your Body

Many of the changes that were initiated in the first trimester of pregnancy now become much more noticeable. You will look obviously pregnant by now, which most women welcome as being infinitely preferable to looking just a little dumpy and overweight. But the changes taking place are not only external; many internal changes (other than the growth of the fetus) are taking place as well.

Uterus At the beginning of this trimester, your uterus will be the size of a large spherical grapefruit. But by the end of this period, the top of the uterus is swelling out just above your navel. Food takes longer to digest now—about twice as long, in fact, as before you were pregnant—so you may feel congested, as if food and baby are competing for space.

Blood Your heart beats more strongly and faster than usual, in order to pump the increased volume of blood around your body and into the placenta. There are more blood vessels in the vagina than before, which will become noticeably dark and soft.

Breasts Your breasts will be much larger now and, if you have not already done so, you should be fitted with a good bra. The nipples and areola will be noticeably darker because of a general increase in pigmentation in the body.

Pigmentation An increase in pigmentation is a characteristic of pregnancy, and tends to affect women in varying degrees, depending on their skin type and coloring.

Women with pale skin will probably notice very little change, whereas olive-skinned women may notice that their skin goes several shades darker everywhere, particularly around the nipples and areola. The genital area also becomes darker.

A dark line down the center of the abdomen, known as the *linea nigra*, usually appears around the fourteenth week. It can be up to 1cm (½in) wide and stretches from the pubic hair to the navel, or, in some women, as far as the breast bone. The *linea nigra* usually fades after delivery. If you have any birthmarks, moles or freckles, these too may darken.

Some women develop blotchy brown patches, called *chloasma*, on the face and neck. These will be made worse by sunlight, so it is best to avoid the sun. Chloasma usually fades after delivery, and disappears completely within around three months.

Stretch Marks During pregnancy you may develop stretch marks on your breasts, abdomen, thighs and buttocks. They develop for two reasons and are certainly not confined to pregnancy.

The first reason is the extra weight and bulk you are putting on causes the collagen bundles of the skin to stretch so much that they tear. And the second is that the increased levels of hormones in the blood disrupt the protein in the skin, making it thinner and more delicate than usual. Stretch marks show as pale wavy stripes on the skin and although they tend to fade a little after delivery, they are permanent and will not disappear altogether.

Prevention is possible, cure is not. Once

stretch marks have appeared, there is nothing you can do to remove them. To help prevent stretch marks from appearing in the first place, it is important to avoid excessive weight gain and to make sure your diet contains plenty of vitamins B, C, E, zinc and silica to help maintain the elasticity of the skin. Massage the skin gently with a good quality oil enriched with vitamin E to help the skin maintain its suppleness. Some essential oils are also useful in preventing stretch marks (see Aromatherapy in Part One). There are also a number of herbal remedies which are helpful in preventing stretch marks (see Herbalism in Part One).

Exercise

Now that the chances of miscarriage are much reduced, this is a good time to start doing relaxation, flexibility and body awareness exercises. All of these will help you greatly in preparation for the birth.

In week fourteen you should therefore enrol in prenatal exercise classes too. A number of organizations and many hospitals hold classes. If you are already practicing yoga, you will know that there are a number of yoga postures which are particularly good for you at this time. Many will help you deal with some of the most common complaints such as backache and constipation (see pages 103–104).

Pelvic Floor Exercises

The hormones of pregnancy prepare the body for delivery by softening the pelvic floor muscles. These muscles support the uterus, bowel and bladder. If pressure from the baby causes the pelvic floor to become weak, this can lead to vague aches and pains, and at worst, to urinary incontinence, and even prolapse of the uterus. Pelvic floor

exercises are recommended in almost every class a pregnant woman might enroll in, and with good reason too. These simple exer-cises will help prevent the pelvic floor from weakening and ultimately will save you a great deal of trouble in the future. Incontinence and a prolapsed womb seem a very high price to pay for not doing these simple exercises.

The muscles of the pelvic floor tighten when you stop the flow of urine. The next time you have to urinate, try stopping mid-flow and you will become aware of these muscles. You can also feel them working if you put a finger into your vagina and squeeze hard.

Picture in your mind a figure eight of muscles around your vagina and urethra above and your rectum below. Tighten these muscles, front and back in turn. Hold them for a few seconds at a time, relaxing in between. Repeat five times. Then finish with a general tightening of the whole area. This simple exercise can be done anywhere and should be done at least a couple of times a day.

Childbirth Classes

Childbirth classes may be run by the hospital, the community health services, or an independent childbirth organization. They usually start at around week twenty-four. Some of these classes are for women only, and some are for couples, the latter being more popular with people who recognize that childbirth is a joint enterprise.

They are valuable for two main reasons; first, you are told what to expect and how best to prepare for labor and delivery, and second, you will have an opportunity to share common problems and feelings with other couples in the same situation as you.

Your Baby

Week fourteen Your baby is fully formed by now. All its vital organs are in place, arms and legs, fingers and toes formed. It is gaining weight fast and will develop in size rather than in structure or form from now on. Its heartbeat is still not audible with a stethoscope but can be heard with a little hand-held electronic device called a Doptone or Doppler. The placenta is in place and is just starting to function.

Week sixteen Your baby is growing very quickly now, gaining in length and is beginning to move around a great deal although you probably will not feel it yet. The baby can turn its head, open its mouth, and move its chest and tummy up and down as if it were breathing deeply. It yawns and stretches. It can frown. There is a growth of fine hair, known as lanugo, all over its body. The placenta is completely formed now. Fetal length is 16cm (6in).

Week eighteen You are probably just beginning to be aware of the baby's movements now, which you experience as very soft ripple-like movements. The baby's arms and legs are well-formed, and the baby does a lot of kicking, bumping, twisting and turning within its amniotic sac. It is able to move quite freely within the sac because it is lying in salt water, which gives it extra buoyancy. The wall of the uterus is springy, so the baby can push against it with its feet, its hands or its head, then bounce off it. Many babies are especially energetic in the evening when their mothers are more relaxed, therefore you are most likely to feel the first signs of life—a little kick—then.

Week twenty At this stage, the baby's head is large in proportion to the rest of its body. The teeth are beginning to form in the jawbone. Hair is growing on its head. You may be very conscious of your baby's movements by now: they feel like fluttering. At around this point the key ultrasound scan is often done and most hospitals recommend it. The baby is checked in all respects and it is an opportunity to look for abnormalities such as spina bifida, kidney, brain and heart defects. Fetal length is 25cm (10in).

Week twenty-four The baby is getting longer and is still very thin. Creases are visible on its palms and fingertips, and its skin is red and wrinkled. Fingernails have formed now. It is sucking its thumb and it may hiccup a lot. The baby is learning to co-ordinate sucking and swallowing in preparation for feeding after the birth. The organs of balance inside the ear have developed and are already the same size as an adult's. The baby's eyes begin to open occasionally but do not remain open yet. It has delicate eyelashes and eyebrows, and can perceive light through the abdominal wall. Even at week twenty-four, it is difficult to hear the heart with a stethoscope. Fetal length is 33cm (13in).

Week twenty-seven The baby's head is now somewhat smaller in comparison with its body; and the baby is beginning to get a little fatter. The whole body is coated with a kind of waxy substance, known as vernix, which prevents its skin from becoming soggy in the amniotic fluid. Fetal length is 37cm (14 ½in).

Your Feelings

By now, there is the sense of having set-tled down into your pregnancy. The chances of miscarriage are greatly reduced, and the early sickness and fatigue have gone, leaving you with a sense of well-being.

During this time you can relax and indulge yourself in the dreams you have for your baby. You obviously want it to be healthy and happy, and we all hope for a world in which our children can grow up safely. Take time to get in touch with those feelings. This is a time when visualization comes into its own, so close your eyes and imagine the baby inside you. Imagine how your own body is nurturing the growing baby. Many mothers feel that their baby is now very real and begin to carry on one-sided conversations. There is some evidence to suggest that babies may learn to recog-nize their mother's voice from the womb.

Communication does not have to be restricted to talking; play music to your baby and carry on an inner conversation. This effort to communicate helps you form a bond with the baby even before it is born, and, even if very little of it penetrates the baby's watery world, it has a profound effect on your emotions and on your psychological readiness for the most important role you are about to assume.

The Father's Role

Your partner will be abundantly aware of your pregnancy by now and will be able to feel the baby's movements when he puts his hand against your abdomen. The first time this happens can be a very exciting experi-ence for him. But it is not unusual for a father-to-be to feel a little removed from the pregnancy at this time. Certainly all the big changes seem to be happening to you and he may feel left out. He may even feel jealous of all the attention that you are get-ting. He could also feel anxious at the prospect of fatherhood, the change it means for him as an individual and the change it will mean for your relationship. It is most important that you discuss these feelings, whether negative or positive, which, if left unspoken and unresolved, may lead to ten-sion in your relationship.

Sex

If you lost interest in sex early on in the pregnancy, as some women who suffer with morning sickness do, it has probably now returned. Some women in fact, feel much more sexual while they are pregnant, find-ing arousal easier and orgasm much more intense. It is possible that the hormones of pregnancy are somewhat responsible, but the general feelings of well-being and hap-piness at this point in your life may make sex a more intense pleasure.

Given your changing shape you may have to experiment with different positions in which to make love. It is certainly a good excuse to abandon the old standard posi-tions for something more exciting—lying flat on your back is not very comfortable at this point. Luxuriate in the sensuality of your changing shape, and allow your part-ner to get to know and appreciate the new ample you! Somehow not having to worry about contraception also seems to loosen inhibitions, leading to more satisfying sex for some couples. Enjoy each other now, for sleepless nights lie ahead.

Prenatal Tests

There are several prenatal tests that you may be offered in the clinic when you go for check-ups during this trimester. Accept only those tests that you feel happy about and do not allow yourself to be persuaded into having any treatment, test or procedure that you do not want.

The Triple AFP Test

This test measures the level of three hormones in the mother's blood: *alphafetoprotein* (AFP), *human chorionic gonadotrophin* (HCG) and *estriol* (ES) and is usually taken between the fifteenth and twenty-second weeks.

At the same time as the blood sample is taken for the triple AFP, a scan measurement will be taken of the fetus, along with the mother's weight. This information will then be fed into a computer and the risk probability will be calculated. This then gives a risk probability (for example, 1 in 400 chance) that the baby might have Down's syndrome. It is not a definite result, only a probability. This test is not a primary test for spina bifida, although if the AFP is high, this could be an indication that spina bifida is a possible problem. A detailed ultrasound scan can provide the necessary information to determine the likelihood of the existence of spina bifida.

If the test is screen positive, then the mother would be counseled to consider having an amniocentesis test, which would be used to gather more genetic material so that chromosomes not examined by the AFP test could be analyzed. This test can determine the likelihood of risk of Down's syndrome.

Amniocentesis

One of the most important prenatal diagnostic tests available to a pregnant woman is amniocentesis, a test used to detect some of the most serious abnormalities in the developing baby including spina bifida and Down's syndrome. In this test, a sample of amniotic fluid is taken out of the womb using a long hollow needle. The needle is passed through the abdominal wall to the amniotic sac. While the procedure is being carried out, the doctor will use ultrasound scan to determine the exact location of the baby and the placenta so that the needle can stay clear of these. Fluid is extracted, then the fluid is spun in a centrifuge, which separates out the cells shed by the baby. These are cultured for two and a half to five weeks.

Amniocentesis is Done if:

- *The obstetrician suspects some abnormality*
- *You have already had an abnormal child*
- *There is a family history of abnormality*
- *You are above a certain age, usually 35*
- *You are a carrier of some hereditary sex-linked disorder, such as muscular dystrophy or hemophilia, in which a male child has a 50/50 chance of inheriting the disease.*

The test gives conclusive evidence as to the child's sex, which is why the test is important in determining the chances of having a baby with a gender-linked disease. Doctors are not willing, however, to perform the test merely to find out if the baby is a boy or a girl. (Some people particularly want either one or the other and would

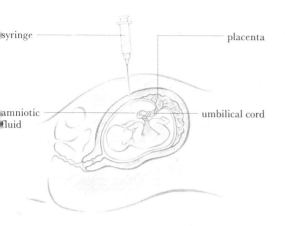

syringe — placenta

amniotic fluid — umbilical cord

Above. In amniocentesis a small sample of amniotic fluid is obtained from the womb using a long hollow needle, which passes through the abdominal wall.

envisage a termination if the fetus was not the sex they wanted: doctors would not offer a termination on these grounds.)

The dilemma posed by amniocentesis is that if it detects a serious abnormality, you have to decide whether or not to terminate the pregnancy. This is obviously a difficult decision, particularly since, by the time you get the results of the test, you would be well into your pregnancy and you will have to undergo a form of labor in order to terminate the pregnancy.

Amniocentesis carries a risk of 1 in 200 of miscarriage in the hands of a skilled operator. The risk can be as high as 1 in 100, depending on background factors.

Fetal Blood Sampling (FBS) or Cordocentesis

This test may be done to check for a disorder which is detectable from a blood sample. Cordocentesis may be done if there is a suspicion that the fetus is anemic or has another kind of blood disease. It may also be used as a quick check to see whether a baby

has Down's syndrome or another genetic abnormality (a chromosome check on cord blood can be done immediately, while cells taken during amniocentesis must be cultured, so it takes weeks to get a result). Cordocentesis can also determine if the fetus has an infection. The procedure involves passing a small needle into the womb to extract blood from the fetus. It is similar to amniocentesis but takes slightly longer. There is a risk of 1 in 100 of miscarriage due to the procedure.

A Difficult Dilemma

All prenatal tests potentially create a profound dilemma for the parents-to-be. At worst, if the likelihood of a severe impairment is indicated, each parent has to decide how to act on the information. Do they have the emotional and financial stability to cope with a handicapped child? These are issues that really need to be addressed before you have a test.

Making Plans for the Birth

You will probably book into the hospital now, if home birth is not your choice. Most deliveries in the United States are by physicians, but midwives are being utilized more often in birthing centers and even hospitals. Do not allow yourself to be persuaded into agreeing to a delivery that is not what you want. Refer to Chapter Two in order to make up your mind about this. Also talk to your midwife, your doctor and your partner.

Arrange to have your chosen therapist with you at the delivery if that is what you want. The birth is becoming a reality now, but there is no need to feel apprehensive. Remember: 97 percent of all pregnancies result in a safe and successful delivery of a healthy baby. Be reassured by that.

Therapies for Common Complaints

The most common complaints during the second three months of pregnancy are similar to those of the first trimester, although morning sickness and fatigue should have passed by now. As mentioned earlier, this trimester is one of blooming good health and a tremendous sense of well-being. You may suffer from a number of minor complaints such as constipation, groin and low back pain, hemorrhoids and varicose veins during this trimester and it is worth trying complementary therapies (see the master chart of Complaints and Therapies on pages 153–154 for the most suitable therapy).

To take best advantage of these complementary therapies, you should have professional treatment. And if you plan to treat yourself at home do at least take some professional guidance before you begin. Some therapies are impossible to administer at home but there are others, however, that can easily be administered as self-help treatments. This applies, in particular, to homeopathy and herbal treatments. If you do not gain relief, you will need to consult an experienced therapist.

Homeopathy

Remember your Tissue Salts program which is outlined in Part One (see pages 31–32). There are also a number of homeopathic remedies for specific ailments and complaints. Constipation, for instance, can be treated with Nux vomica 6 taken hourly for up to six doses, or Nux vomica 30 may be taken every three hours for up to six doses. In either case you should discontinue treatment as soon as you feel any change, either physical or emotional.

Herbal Treatment

Similarly, there are several herbal treatments you can try to relieve some of the most common complaints that are likely to affect you in the second three months of pregnancy. Perhaps the easiest conditions to treat yourself include backache, constipation, heartburn, insomnia, thrush and varicose veins. For varicose veins you might try steeping calendula in distilled witch hazel for an hour, then externally applying this solution to the affected area with a wash cloth or cotton wool two or three times daily. An internal remedy for the same complaint is an infusion or decoction of yarrow or St John's wort, drink a wine-glassful two or three times daily (see Herbalism in Part One for further remedies and instructions on preparing infusions or decoctions).

Yoga

Some of the common complaints in pregnancy during this second trimester can be relieved by certain yoga poses. Backache, for example, which is probably the most common complaint of all, not only during the pregnancy itself but for some months after delivery, can be helped by the pelvic tilt. Varicose veins and hemorrhoids, both caused by additional pressure on the veins, can be relieved by practicing leg lifts (see page 72) and legs up against the wall (see page 114). Constipation can be eased with the thunderbolt pose (see page 104).

Backache

Pelvic Tilt This posture relieves the pressure of the fetus on the nerves and blood vessels of the lower pelvis and the upper thighs. It is an excellent posture for relieving backache and improving spinal flexibility. Practice the pelvic tilt daily from now until the end of your pregnancy.

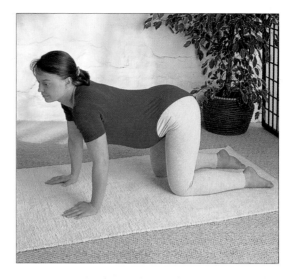

1 *Kneel on all fours and place your hands on the floor beneath your shoulders, shoulder-width apart (right). Both the hands and knees should be square, in order to provide a firm base, and the body and head should both be parallel to the floor.*

2 *As you breathe out, slowly rock backward and sink back on to your feet with your arms stretched out in front of you (see inset, below). Let your head drop forward and your spine relax.*

3 *As you breathe in, gently rock forward, bringing the weight over your arms and hands (below). Continue rocking slowly back and forth as long as feels comfortable. Then slowly sit upright and rest for a moment.*

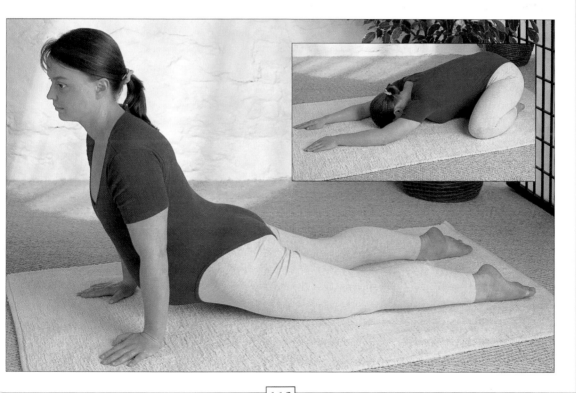

Varicose Veins, Hemorrhoids and Tension

Legs Up Against the Wall This is an excellent posture for relieving varicose veins and hemorrhoids, as it releases any pressure or tension, and reduces swelling. It is also a generally relaxing pose. It is good, too, for strengthening the perineum, in preparation for birth.

You may find this position uncomfortable if you are on a hard floor; try lying on a rug and supporting your head with a cushion.

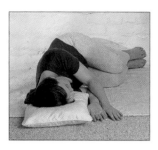

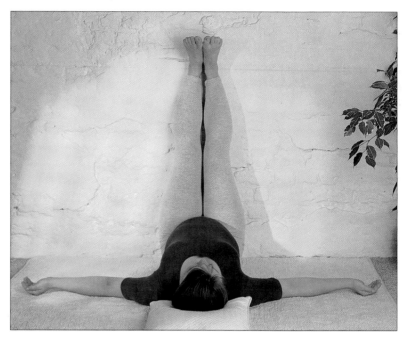

1 *Lie on your side, with your bottom against the wall.*

2 *Roll on to your back and lift your legs straight up, so that they are flat against the wall. Your arms should be straight out on either side, palms facing upward. Lie like that for a few minutes.*

3 *Move your legs as far apart as they will go without straining. Lie like that for a few minutes.*

4 *Alternatively, bend your knees. Then straighten them, roll on to your side and rest before rising.*

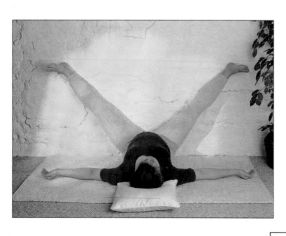

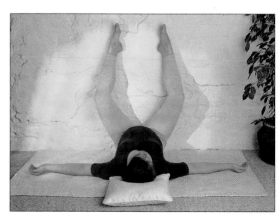

Stress and Tension

Relaxation The room should be warm, dimly-light and quiet. You may want to lie on a blanket and place a small pillow under your head. Cover yourself with a light blanket if you want.

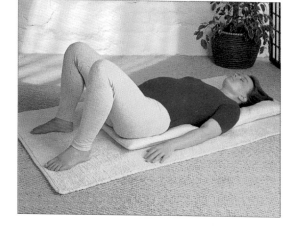

1 *Lie down, with arms at your sides, palms facing upward, legs slightly apart (right). Close your eyes. In the later stages of pregnancy, you can lie on one side, with one knee drawn up toward the chest (below). Support your head, your stomach and your knee with cushions.*

2 *Take a deep breath and relax completely. Mentally go through each part of your body, starting at the toes and working up through the whole body. Release any tension you feel by breathing into the tension and letting it go.*

3 *Your whole body will be relaxed and feeling heavy, sinking into the floor. Bring your attention to your breathing, watch the natural flow of your breath as it enters and leaves your body. Let your mind relax for five to ten minutes, focusing on the flow of your breath.*

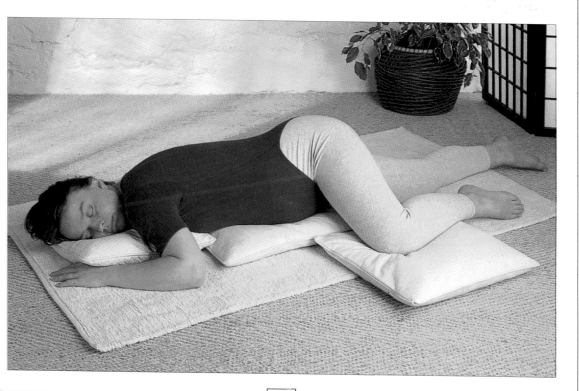

CHAPTER FOUR

The Last Three Months

~

During the last term of pregnancy, from weeks twenty-eight to forty, you may begin to feel that you have been pregnant forever! You may be feeling increasingly tired through sleeplessness, and may even feel breathless on any kind of exertion. Do not do any more than you feel comfortable with now, though gentle exercise may help you relax.

This is a time when you should pamper yourself and take it easy. Make sure that you are getting plenty of rest and as much sleep as you can. Your sleep may be interrupted frequently now with trips to the lavatory, kicks from the baby, and a difficulty in finding a comfortable position, so take short naps when you can during the day to compensate for any lost sleep at night. This is excellent preparation for the time after the birth when any prolonged period of sleep may seem like a far-off luxury.

By now, the skin on your abdomen will have become very thin and stretched, and stretch marks—if you have them—will be obvious. You will visit your prenatal clinic every two weeks from now until week thirty-six; from then until delivery your visits will be weekly.

Your Body

By now your pregnancy is obvious for all the world to see; your stomach will be significantly bigger and you may find that clothes bought in the earlier stages of pregnancy no longer fit. During this last trimester, your body is adjusting to a rapidly growing baby and preparing itself for the coming labor.

The Uterus In the early months of pregnancy, the developing baby was easily accommodated in the space within the growing uterus. During the second trimester, the narrow area between the cavity of the uterus and the cervix, known as the isthmus, enlarges, giving the baby more space. This part of the uterus is known as the lower segment.

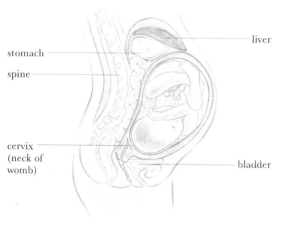

stomach

spine

liver

cervix
(neck of
womb)

bladder

Above. *The baby's increasing size exerts pressure on the bladder, the neck of the womb and the spine.*

As the uterus rises and both uterus and baby push up under your diaphragm and ribs, you may feel sore on the lower edge of the ribcage. Your navel will have flattened out by now. By week thirty-six or so, the heavy uterus, pressing on a large blood vessel behind it, slows down the flow of blood back to your heart when you are lying down; this may make you feel nauseous and giddy. Many women find it easier to lie on their side, or at least well propped up.

Braxton Hicks Contractions The uterine muscles undergo weak contractions throughout pregnancy. They are so weak and short-lived that you may not even notice them in the early months, though by now if you put a hand on your abdomen you will probably feel the muscles going tight and hard.

These painless "practice" contractions, known as Braxton Hicks contractions, occur every 20 minutes and last about 60 seconds. They are important because they help uterine growth, as well as ensuring a good circulation of blood through the uterus.

In the last month of pregnancy, Braxton Hicks contractions may become quite noticeable. They feel like firm squeezes of the tummy and can become so strong that they make you catch your breath and can sometimes be mistaken for labor. The cervix is usually strong and tight enough to withstand Braxton Hicks contractions. You should try rehearsing your breathing and relaxation exercises with Braxton Hicks contractions as soon as they become lengthy and strong.

Backache Backache can become more pronounced now. Pregnancy hormones have softened the ligaments attached to your pelvis so that a large baby will be able to pass through a relatively small pelvis. It is the stretching of these ligaments that can cause backache. There are various yoga poses that can help relieve the nagging ache (*see pages 103, 113 and 126*). A soothing massage from your partner can also work wonders. You may find low-heeled or flat shoes more comfortable, and these are certainly better for your back and your general posture.

Fatigue Feeling tired is an inescapable part of childbearing, particularly during the first two or three months of pregnancy, the last couple of months before the baby is born and also for several months after you have given birth. Set yourself a routine of early nights whenever you can and, if you know you will be having a late night, then try to snatch a half-hour rest before you go out.

Breasts Colostrum—the first milk, especially rich in vitamins, minerals and protein—may begin to leak from your breasts. Secretion of colostrum is caused by one of the hormones of pregnancy, known as *human placental lactogen* (HPL) and indicates that the placenta is functioning well and nourishing the baby. You may need to wear breast pads to contain leaks. If you are planning to breastfeed, now is the time to begin preparing your nipples. While bathing or showering, try rubbing them with a wash cloth, and apply comfrey ointment or calendula cream, or buttermilk and honey to keep them supple.

Pigmentation Any changes in pigmentation that you have already noticed are likely to be exaggerated now. The *linea nigra* will probably be clearly visible running down the center of your abdomen.

Itching You may feel a need to scratch your skin, particularly on the stomach itself and sometimes on old stretch marks. This can be alleviated by wearing loose, soft clothing and applying Calamine lotion. If itching is more severe or widespread it can rarely indicate a potentially serious liver complication: Obstetric Cholestasis. If this situation develops, especially with slight yellowing of the eyes, light-colored stools or dark urine, you must see your specialist. Untreated cholestasis leads to serious risks for the mother and her unborn child.

Other Changes Any kind of exertion may make you feel breathless, although breathing problems should ease once your baby's head is engaged—that is, when it drops into the pelvis in preparation for birth. When the baby's head engages, it causes an increase in pressure on the bladder, and is likely to cause a corresponding increase in desire to pass urine. You may also feel a corresponding pain in the pelvic area.

Indigestion may become a problem simply because what you eat competes with the baby for space. Your stomach also empties more slowly, which may mean that a heavy meal leaves you feeling bloated. If this is a problem for you, eat little and often, and incorporate plenty of fiber in your diet. It is important to keep up your intake of calcium-rich foods such as dairy products, particularly if you are suffering from cramps.

Vaginal discharge is common at this time, and may be heavy enough to require you to wear light, stick-on sanitary napkins. Do not use internal tampons. You might begin to massage the perineum to aid elasticity in readiness for the birth. Try massaging the perineum with wheatgerm oil mixed with a few drops of lavender oil. While massaging you can work around the outer walls of the vagina to help them stretch easily.

Your Baby

Week twenty-eight If your baby is born at this point there is a fair chance that it will survive with the help of medical technology. In fact it has been considered legally viable since week twenty-four. This means that if your baby was born now and died, the birth would be registered as a stillbirth rather than a miscarriage. The baby would have breathing difficulties, due to the lack of surfactant in the lungs, and the lack of body fat would mean that the baby would have difficulties regulating its own body temperature.

The baby will have filled up almost all the available room in the uterus, and many babies turn head down at this stage. You will certainly feel a good deal of kicking and fluttering of feet and hands at this stage of your pregnancy. Many babies have particular periods of activity which seem to be consistent from day to day and often correspond to the times during the day when their mothers are resting.

Week thirty-two The baby is perfectly formed by now. Its lungs are developed, which means that if it were to be born now, it would have a good chance of survival. The baby's movements can be clearly felt. At this point it will probably have turned head down in a cephalic or vertex presentation (*see page 120*). The placenta is mature.

Week thirty-six If this is your first baby, the head will soon engage. Your baby is becoming steadily plumper and is gaining about 14g (½oz) of fat under the skin every day. This will ensure that the baby has an efficient system for regulating heat and cold once it is outside the controlled environment of the uterus. The irises of its eyes are blue. Fingers and toes have developed soft nails which reach right to the ends. Hair on its head may be as long as 2.5cm (1in). The umbilical cord is about 51cm (20in) long and is very slippery, so that although the baby may move around a great deal, including moving through a loop of cord, it is unlikely to form into a tight knot. Fetal length is 46cm (18in).

Week thirty-eight The baby's nervous system is maturing ready for birth. The layer of fat under its skin is now ready to regulate the body temperature when it is born. The lungs are lined with surfactant, which resembles bubbles of foam. This will keep the lungs partially inflated each time the baby breathes out after it is born. Without surfactant the lungs would collapse. The baby's heartbeat is about twice as fast as yours, about 110–150 beats per minute. Your partner may be able to hear the baby's heartbeat simply by putting his ear against your tummy.

Week forty The baby's movements decrease as there is less space inside the uterus. You may miss these movements which have become so much a part of your life. However, you may still feel strong kicks from the baby's hands and feet. In a boy, the testicles will have descended. When the baby is awake, its eyes are open a good deal of the time. The baby is able to discern light through the uterine wall and can feel vibration made by sound, as well as associating certain sounds with the mood of mother. Fetal length is 51cm (20in).

The Baby's Position

In most cases, the baby will have turned head down in a *cephalic* or *vertex* presentation by week thirty-two, and this is the best position for birth. It tips head down partly because its head is the heaviest part of its body and partly so that its weight can stimulate the processes of labor. Most babies turn facing head down some time after week twenty-eight and then stay that way until they are born, though a small baby who has plenty of space in the uterus may still change position several times over the next few weeks.

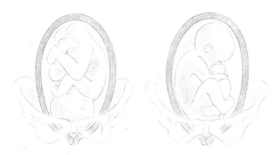

Positions at Birth
Above left. *Head-down presentation, ready for birth.*
Above right. *Typical breech (head-up) presentation.*

A few babies remain in the head-up position in the uterus for a little longer and a minority of babies remain head-up and are born this way, which is known as *breech* presentation. You should know when your baby is in the head-down position because you will feel the baby's feet kicking against your ribs, rather than the hard ball of the baby's head. You may also feel the baby's head bouncing against your springy pelvic floor muscles. To start with, the baby will do this gently and, as it drops further into your pelvis, it will do so more vigorously.

Turning the Baby

If your baby is the breech position, your doctor may want to try and turn it round, using a technique known as external version. This entails a gentle massage of the abdomen. It is no longer done automatically though, and some physicians prefer not to try it. It is not attempted before week thirty-six, in case the baby decides to turn itself, so there is no need to be concerned too soon.

What You Can Do

You may be able to encourage the baby to turn itself around using the following exercise. Lie on your back with your hips raised on a sofa or a stack of pillows, and your head and shoulders on the floor. Stay like this for twenty minutes at a time if you can stand it, and do it two or three times a day. This position may encourage the baby to turn itself. Take advantage of the time to relax; put some music on and flip through some magazines if you feel like it.

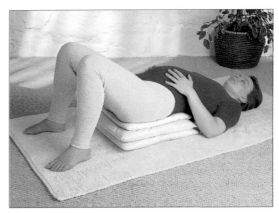

Above. *Lie with your hips raised on a pile of cushions above your head and shoulders in order to encourage your baby to turn head down.*

Complementary Therapies

Several complementary therapies claim to be able to help turn the baby around. An acupuncturist may use moxibustion (the application of heat to the skin by burning a specially prepared herb), or the therapist may insert needles to a point on the outer edge of the little toe to encourage a breech baby to turn. Similarly, a shiatsu practitioner can apply pressure here. Therapists may recommend that you do the earlier mentioned exercise (see page 120) regularly while they are treating you. Once the baby has turned, squat regularly in order to encourage the baby's head to engage.

The homeopathic remedy Pulsatilla has a reputation for turning breech babies in a large number of cases. However, it is best to be treated constitutionally by a trained homeopath.

Your Feelings

The nesting instinct may become increasingly strong around this time and you may find yourself overwhelmed by strange urges to clean your home or re-decorate. Try to keep your level of activity within reason—washing all the walls in the nursery a week before the baby is due is not necessarily the best way to rest and prepare for the delivery. This urge is very common, however, in women in late pregnancy.

You may feel quite calm most of the time about the approaching birth, yet most women also have moments of panic. Will I be able to cope with the pain? What will they do to me? Will the baby be all right? Will I be a good mother? Will the baby have an effect on our relationship? These are all common anxieties. A woman's feelings at this time can best be described as a mixture of excitement interspersed with moments of fear. The fear commonly floods in at nighttime, when you cannot sleep and you feel alone.

It may be reassuring to know that these strong emotions are a way of helping you prepare yourself for all the changes ahead. Heightened sensitivity and the ease with which tears often flow are all signs that you are in an emotional state that will make you particularly responsive to your newborn baby when it finally arrives.

By week thirty-six many women start to feel that they have been pregnant for long enough. They would like to get on with things—to see the baby and to hold it in their arms. They may feel tired, fed up, huge and impatient.

By week forty, when the expected date of delivery arrives and perhaps passes, you may become anxious. Remember that only five percent of all babies arrive on the due date, and it is not at all unusual for babies, particularly first babies, to arrive later than predicted. Although pregnancy is calculated as forty weeks, this is by no means set in stone. It could be thirty-eight weeks or forty-two weeks. Not everyone is sure of their conception date, so the delivery date will be uncertain too.

You will probably have discussed the possibility of late arrival with your hospital and, if so, you will know the hospital's policy on induction. You will no doubt have formed a view on this yourself and will have passed this on, through your birth plan, to the people who are looking after you.

Communicating with Your Baby

As your pregnancy advances you will become more and more aware of all the different parts of your baby. You will be able to identify its feet, its head, its curved back and its rounded bottom. Getting to know your baby and its various bits of anatomy in this way is greatly reassuring. You can point out the various parts of your baby's body to your partner, who will no doubt take great pleasure in discovering for himself the fact that the stomach actually conceals a real baby.

The Father-to-be

No matter how excited he is, it is by no means unusual for a prospective father to be a little apprehensive at this time. He may worry about how good a father he is going to be. He may be anxious about the pain his partner is likely to feel when she gives birth. These are all quite normal feelings and he may find it helpful to talk to friends who are already fathers. Some prenatal classes run a fathers-only evening, which usually includes a film of a delivery, then a discussion of the general procedures which are used in that particular hospital. It includes advice on how to help the laboring mother, what to expect in the delivery room as well as advice on coping with feeling nervous, frightened and faint, and all the other fears facing prospective fathers.

Preparing for the Birth

There are a number of things you will do during this last trimester of pregnancy which will help you prepare for labor and for the birth itself. Making a birth plan, attending parenting classes, various routine hospital checks and finally packing your case if you are having a hospital birth, or setting aside the things required if you are having a home birth, are important considerations now.

Making a Birth Plan

Your birth plan should outline in writing all your wishes regarding your labor and the delivery of your baby. It is best if you discuss all your wishes in advance with the people who are caring for you, rather than just hand the list to them. A copy of your birth plan will then be inserted in your records.

If you are being cared for by the same people throughout pregnancy and labor, a birth plan is probably not necessary, because they will be familiar with your wishes and feelings. However, if there are likely to be people at the birth whom you do not know and who therefore do not know exactly what your wishes are, a birth plan is a good idea.

Questions you might like to address in your birth plan include your views on being shaved (not usually done nowadays), continuous fetal monitoring, having your water broken, oxytocin (a hormone used to speed up labor), intravenous drips, types of pain relief, induction, episiotomy, cesarean delivery and forceps delivery.

All these issues should be discussed with your doctor or midwife first. They have considerably more experience of childbirth than you and they can share this with you to your benefit. Discuss the advantages and disadvantages of all the various procedures with them and record your feelings in your birth plan.

You might also like to consider who you want to be with you during labor (your partner, a therapist of your choice), and record it on your birth plan. You can also stipulate what you would like to have with you in the birthing room (a bean bag or mat, dim lights, music, aromatherapy oils, herbs). Other considerations for your birth plan include things you would like to do: be free to move around; be kept fully informed and party to any decisions that are made; and what position you would like to assume for delivery. It can also include what you would like to do after the birth: whether you are planning to breastfeed; whether you want to be woken at night to feed your baby yourself; where you want your baby to sleep; and how long you are likely to remain in hospital.

Parenting Classes

You will be able to attend parenting classes at around week thirty-two of your pregnancy. These classes are usually designed for both parents to attend together, though some mothers come on their own. Parenting classes are available at most hospitals and also at various mother and baby groups. It is worth shopping around to make sure that you choose the classes that concentrate on the aspects of pregnancy and child care which you find most compelling.

The classes are designed to give parents information about the practical and emotional aspects of pregnancy, the birth and the handling of their new baby, as well as the all-important confidence to cope at each stage. Parenting classes provide the opportunity to ask all those questions that you would have liked to ask during your visits to the prenatal clinic but never had time for. They are aimed in particular at first-time parents, though many second attend to refresh their memor if there has been a long gap sin baby. The classes should give yo standing of what happens du nancy, labor and birth, as well as techniques of relaxation, breath..ng and exercise, all of which will help prepare you for labor.

Any good class will also offer valuable information to help you cope with a tiny baby, as well as addressing issues such as breastfeeding, diapers, crying babies, and how to recognize illness.

Routine Hospital Checks

During the last month of pregnancy, you will probably have weekly prenatal checks during which routine tests for high blood pressure and pre-eclampsia will be done.

If your blood pressure rises in late pregnancy, your heart cannot pump blood efficiently around your body and this means that your baby may not be receiving enough nourishment or oxygen. This may mean, in turn, that the baby could be smaller than it otherwise would have been, and that it may become distressed during labor. High blood pressure can be brought down by drugs, which do no harm to the baby.

High blood pressure, together with swelling of the ankles and hands, and protein in the urine, are also some of the signs of pre-eclampsia. This is a condition that can be life-threatening to both mother and baby if undetected. A woman with pre-eclampsia may need to be admitted to hospital for medical observation. If routine tests indicate that there is anything wrong, other tests may be carried out, including ultrasound scans and fetal heart monitoring done by placing a belt round the mother's ɔmen. If pre-eclampsia is diagnosed sometimes early delivery, either by induction or by cesarean section, becomes necessary in order to safeguard the lives of the mother and the baby.

Preparing for Delivery Day

The impending birth will be at the forefront of your mind a great deal of the time now, and it is as well to be prepared for it in case you should go into labor sooner than you expect. If you are having your baby in hospital, pack your hospital bag a few weeks before your baby is due. Check with the hospital to find out what they provide—usually diapers and the baby's clothing during your stay—as this is likely to vary considerably from area to area.

Pack your bag in readiness for an unexpected departure. As you already know, babies do not necessarily arrive on schedule and many are a little early or late. At the onset of labor you do not want to have to worry about finding clean clothes and toiletries before you can leave for the hospital.

There are a number of things which you may wish to take with you to help make you more comfortable throughout your labor and delivery. You may find a water spray and facecloth or sponge to wipe your face very refreshing if you become very hot during your labor. Lip salve for chapped lips may also be quite useful. Pack a hot-water bottle in case you have backache, and warm socks in case your legs start to tremble with fatigue during labor.

You may also like to take mineral water and fruit juice in case you are thirsty. (Check that the hospital allows you to drink during labor. Some may not, especially if there is a risk of having to have an emergency cesarean section.) Pack a mirror so that you can watch your baby being born. Also include any homeopathic and herbal remedies that you have planned to use for pain relief, and take massage oils or talcum powder for massage during labor.

For the rest of your hospital stay, you may find you need two or three front-opening nightdresses if you plan to breastfeed, a bathrobe, slippers, nursing bras and sanitary napkins. Obviously, you will want to take your ordinary toiletries and cosmetics. You may also find a telephone card or a good stock of coins and your address book useful, as well as writing materials and books and magazines.

Preparing for a Home Delivery

If you are having a home delivery, you will have discussed the requirements for the birth with your midwife. She will be responsible for all of the medical equipment and supplies necessary, and will bring these with her when your labor starts.

However there are a number of things you may need to prepare yourself for a comfortable and safe home delivery. These may include some of the items listed above, in particular any remedies which you might be planning to use, such as water and juices, sprays, massage oils and the like.

But you will also need to have a number of other things on hand including clean sheets and towels, preferably old ones so that it will not matter if they are stained, a telephone, a chair, several large cushions, a large bean bag and perhaps a low stool. The midwife will also need an adequate source of light, perhaps a flexible lamp, for close examination. The room in which you plan to give birth should be adequately heated to at least around 21 degrees C (70 degrees F).

Therapies for Common Complaints

The most common complaints during the final three months of pregnancy include the ever-present backache, abdominal pain, breathlessness, dizziness, leg cramps, insomnia, edema and swelling of hands, legs and ankles. There are a number of complementary therapies that can provide some relief for these complaints.

Relaxation

It is important now to make time for yourself alone and to use it for relaxation. This will bring a general sense of well-being to both your mind and your body. Focus your thoughts on the baby inside you and on how you will soon give birth.

Relaxation can be used to great benefit in childbirth. These benefits include feeling less pain, being able to conserve energy, feeling more confident, your cervix opening more smoothly, your uterus working better; and feeling less tired after the delivery.

Try the following relaxation exercise in a quiet moment. Also refer to *Meditation* in Part One. Before you begin, make sure that you will not be disturbed for twenty minutes or so. Begin by sitting, supported by cushions or pillows in any position that feels comfortable. Make sure that your neck and the small of your back are well supported. Drop your head forward slightly and close your eyes, then pull your shoulders down and concentrate on your breathing which should be slow and easy.

Now concentrate on each part of your body in turn, starting with your feet, then legs and so on until you have worked through your whole body. Feel each part relax in turn and allow any muscular tension to be released. Now focus on your breath as it enters and leaves your body. Stay like this for three or four minutes.

You could also ask your partner to give you a gentle abdominal or lower back massage with geranium oil diluted in a carrier oil (*see* Aromatherapy *on page 48*).

Homeopathy

In addition to your Tissue Salts program (*see pages 31–32*) there are a number of remedies for complaints common to this trimester. Consult a homeopath for specific complaints and take the dosages recommended. Edema, dizziness and cramps respond to homeopathic treatment.

Herbal Treatment

There are several herbal treatments that you can try to relieve some of the common complaints that are likely to affect you now. Some conditions you can treat yourself include cramps, heartburn, fluid retention, varicose veins and hemorrhoids. Fluid retention can be treated with a cupful of infusion of either corn silk, horsetail or dandelion leaves taken three times daily (*see* Herbalism *on page 26*).

Yoga

Some of the common complaints of this trimester can be relieved by yoga poses. Backache, for example, can be helped by the frog posture, pelvic discomfort by the moon pose, and edema by leg lifts.

Backache

Frog Pose This posture is particularly recommended for relieving backache. The uterus should rest comfortably on the floor between your knees.

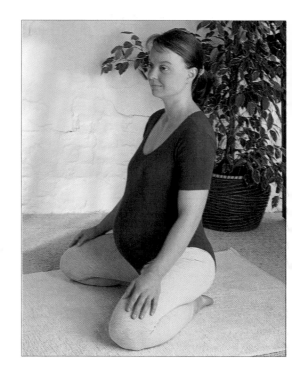

1 *Sit on your heels or between your feet (right). Knees should be spread apart as wide as is comfortable.*

2 *Lower your body forward toward the floor (inset, below). Keep your back as straight as possible, using a pillow to lean on if needed. Rest arms on the floor.*

3 *Now raise your buttocks into the air as high as you can (below). Hold them there and then lower them back down again. Rest for a moment and then repeat. Do this as many times as feels comfortable.*

When you are ready, stretch your arms out in front of you and lift up slowly into a sitting position. Rest there for a few moments before getting up.

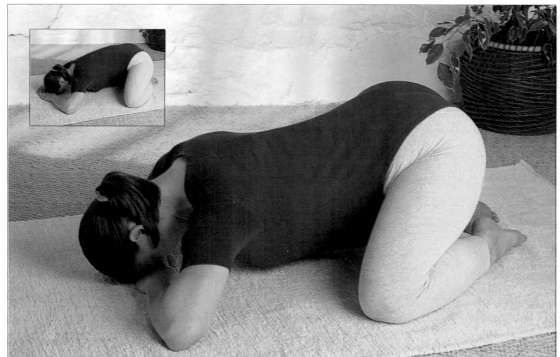

Pelvic Discomfort

Moon Pose This position is particularly good for any pelvic discomfort which you may feel once the baby's head is engaged. Begin this excercise by kneeling up, with your feet stretched backward. Then follow the sequence laid out below.

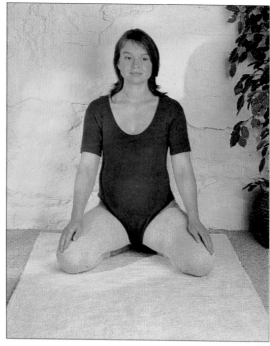

1 *Sit down on to your feet with your feet stretched backward and your big toes crossed (right). Your knees should be together and your heels apart. Lower your buttocks on to the insides of your feet, with the heels on the sides of the hips. Place your hands on your knees, palms facing downward.*

2 *As you inhale, raise your arms vertically above your head (below), stretching your torso upward as far as is comfortable for you.*

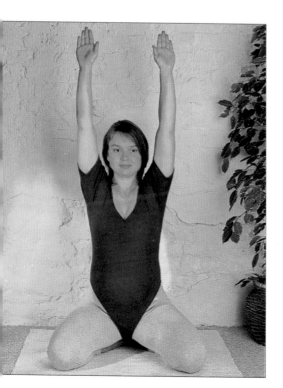

3 *As you exhale, bend your trunk forward, opening the knees enough to accommodate your stomach (below), and keeping your arms stretched in front of you. If you can, rest hands and forehead on the floor. Breathe normally and stay in this position for a few minutes.*

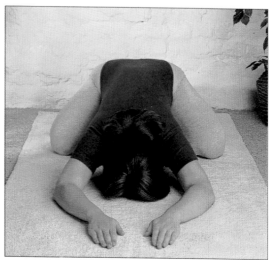

CHAPTER FIVE

Giving Birth

❧

After forty weeks of pregnancy you are about to give birth to your long-awaited baby. Seeing and holding your baby after what seems like an endless wait is the fulfilment of the dream begun by you and your partner. The prospect of seeing your baby will make the apprehension you may be feeling about labor a little more bearable. You are obviously hoping for a good labor—not necessarily one that is entirely pain-free as that may not be realistic, but at least a relaxed and stress-free one with your own precious and healthy baby to rejoice over at the end of it. You will know that when your labor starts, you have done everything in your power to achieve a stress-free delivery, including giving up smoking, cutting out alcohol, exercising regularly, eating properly and making sure that you are well rested. Everything is in place for the arrival of your baby.

Your Feelings

By the end of your pregnancy you will probably be looking forward to giving birth and holding your baby in your arms at last. You may feel that you have been pregnant all your life and you have had enough. You cannot wait to have it over with. At the same time, though, and especially if this is your first baby or if your previous experience of childbirth was at all difficult, you may be feeling a little apprehensive. What kind of labor will you have? Will it be easy or will it be dreadfully painful? Will you be able to cope with it without letting yourself down? Will you lose control? These are all questions that may be running through your mind at the moment.

Although fear and anxiety are entirely natural at this time, it is usual for these feelings to be overtaken by a great excitement as the moment when the baby will be born approaches. In the last few days before the birth, it is common for feelings of fear and apprehension to be replaced by a quiet energy, confidence and optimism.

The Father

Becoming a father is a momentous event, especially if it is for the first time. The father-to-be will anticipate seeing, touching and hearing his new baby. If he chooses to be present at the child's birth, it is likely to be one of the most powerful and moving experiences of his life, one that he will never forget.

As recently as the 1970s, it was still unusual for a man to attend the birth of his child, especially if this took place in hospital. Now, however, it is the rule rather than the exception; most women want their partner's support during the birth of their children, and most fathers want to be there.

There are some fathers who do not wish to be present at the birth of their children, and their feelings should be respected. There are also some mothers who do not want their partner to be there, either because they feel a strong need to be alone at such an important time in their lives, or because they do not want to be seen at such a vulnerable and private time. Their feelings, too, should be respected. No one should be persuaded to go against what they know is right for them.

Advice to the Father

There are a number of things that you can do to help your partner during labor. You should, above all, remember that labor can be a traumatic and difficult time for a woman, and therefore be prepared to deal with any demands and perhaps even aggressive behavior that she may display. Do not be put off by it.

You should try to help her to relax, particularly between contractions so that she conserves her strength. Encourage her by telling her she is doing fine, and certainly never criticize her. Be alert to her moods and try to fit in with them.

If she says she wants to push or she starts to grunt and make pushing motions, tell the midwife. Once the midwife has told her that she is fully dilated and she can push, let the midwife guide her through the pushing stage. Your role is a supportive one now rather than an active one. Needless to say, always be guided by the midwife even if it is not clear to you what is happening.

Your Baby

By the time your baby is born, you will have been pregnant for some thirty-eight weeks. Pregnancy is always calculated as forty weeks because it is counted from the date of your last period, but in fact, gestation usually lasts for thirty-eight weeks.

Week forty The baby is prepared for birth. It has practiced breathing movements, sucking and swallowing in anticipation of life in the outside world. It has mastered a whole range of physical reflexes which allow it to grasp tightly, lift and turn its head, make stepping movements, blink and close its eyes, and respond once it has made its appearance in the world, to stimuli such as touch, smell, light and sound. An average full-term baby can measure between 45–55cm (18–22in) and can weigh anything from 2.9–5kg (6–11 lb).

The Stages of Labor

The process of birth consists of three continuous stages. During the first stage the uterus begins to contract at regular intervals until the cervix (neck of the uterus) opens, or dilates, to about 10cm (4in) in diameter. Until then it is not possible for the baby's head to pass through. This stage is usually the longest part of labor.

The second stage begins when the cervix is fully dilated and ends with the passage of the baby through the cervix and pelvic canal, through the vagina—in other words, the birth of the baby. The second stage is generally much shorter than the first stage.

The third stage, which follows the birth of the baby, occurs when the placenta separates from the lining of the uterus and further contractions expel it from the uterus.

Pain in Labor

Individual women experience the pain of labor with different intensities. In early labor the contractions are often likened to menstrual cramps and sometimes they entail nothing more than a mild backache.

Some women feel a sharp wave of pain right across their abdomen, which reaches its height for a few seconds and then subsides. At the same time, they can feel a severe tightening and hardening of the uterine muscle which lasts for a few seconds, before the muscle relaxes again. Contractions vary quite considerably in length and strength. At their worst, they can follow one another relentlessly, which is not only painful but also exhausting, not allowing the mother to catch her breath and breathe into the next contraction.

How Long Does Labor Last?

The length of labor can vary considerably. In general, first-birth labors tend to be longer, while second and subsequent ones tend to be shorter and may also be easier. The length of labor does not necessarily mean that it is more or less easy or difficult. Contrary to what some people imagine, a short labor can actually be very painful and difficult, while a long one can sometimes be easy.

How Will You Know When Labor Has Started

Many women worry about whether or not they will be able to recognize the signs of impending labor. They may be anxious about giving birth on a bus or in a taxi. This is a common anxiety, but it happens very rarely. There are several important signs that indicate that your labor is starting. These include a "show," which is a discharge of pinkish blood, indicating that the gelatinous plug of mucus that has been blocking the cervical canal during pregnancy has been dislodged and that the cervix is beginning to stretch.

Another good indication is when your water breaks. This painless leakage of amniotic fluid, which can vary from a slight dribble to a heavy gush, indicates that the membranes surrounding the baby in the uterus have ruptured. A further sign is the onset of regular, pronounced contractions.

It is possible for all three signs of labor to occur independently of each other, or in combination. A show and your water breaking are both clear signs that labor is imminent. Together, these cannot be mistaken. If your water breaks, you should be taken to hospital straight away because of the risk of infection. Contractions, on the other hand, can be misleading; some may be Braxton Hicks contractions.

False Labor

All the way through pregnancy, you may feel uterine or Braxton Hicks contractions—a sense of tightening in the abdominal area. In the last weeks of pregnancy, these contractions may become more pronounced and can sometimes be painful. Some women mistake Braxton Hicks for signs of early labor, particularly if this is their first baby. It is important, therefore, to try to distinguish between false labor, which is characterized by Braxton Hicks contractions, and true labor. Braxton Hicks contractions are irregular and do not cause the cervix (neck of the uterus) to dilate. They may occur every twenty minutes or so and last for about twenty or thirty seconds. The contractions of labor, on the other hand, are regular (every ten minutes or so) and cause the cervix to dilate. They last for forty seconds or more.

Time your contractions over an hour. If they get closer together and last longer in duration each time, you are probably in labor. If you are in any doubt, you should ring the hospital and talk to someone on the labor ward. They may advise you to come in to be examined, where they will be able to tell immediately whether you are in labor by looking at your cervix. If it is not dilated, you are not in labor. If it is, your labor has begun.

Going to Hospital

The process of labor and birth will be the same, whether you have your baby in hospital or at home. The procedure, however, will be quite different.

Some women delay going to hospital for as long as possible in the belief that this will save them long, boring hours in the labor ward and that medical assistance and monitoring will be reduced to a minimum. There is probably something to be said for the first reason, but the second is less sound. If someone needs medical assistance, they will either receive it in a relaxed atmosphere when there is plenty of time, or as a rushed emergency procedure. No one wants to be admitted to hospital and then discharged because they are too early. But doctors agree that a few false alarms are preferable to a lot of last-minute admissions in which the baby arrives within minutes of the mother walking through the doors of the hospital. If in doubt, telephone. They will be sympathetic and they will be able to advise you on the strength of what you can tell them.

Admission to Hospital

When you arrive at the hospital, you will go through the normal admissions procedure, then be taken to the labor ward. Your pulse, temperature and blood pressure will be taken and you will be examined externally and possibly internally in order to judge the baby's position and to see how far the cervix has dilated.

Staying at Home

If you have arranged to have your baby at home, you will not be bound by hospital routine. You will have had the opportunity to get to know your midwife well before the birth, and will have discussed your wishes with her beforehand. When labor starts, you will contact your midwife and you will stay in touch with her by telephone until labor is well established and it is time for her to join you. She will bring all the necessary medical supplies and equipment with her but there are a number of things which you should prepare beforehand (*see photograph right*) including clean sheets, towels, telephone, lamp, chair, low stool, cushions and bean bag, mineral water or juice, a natural sponge, a clean nightdress and any remedies you have decided to take.

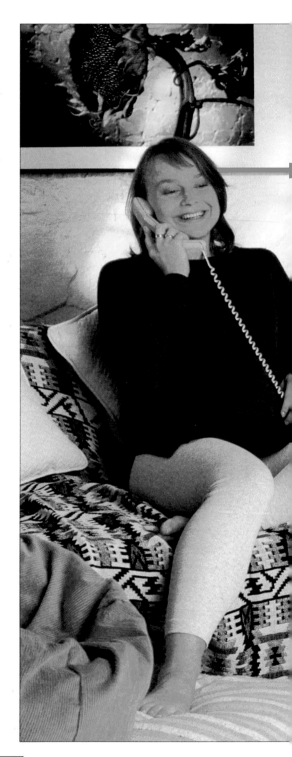

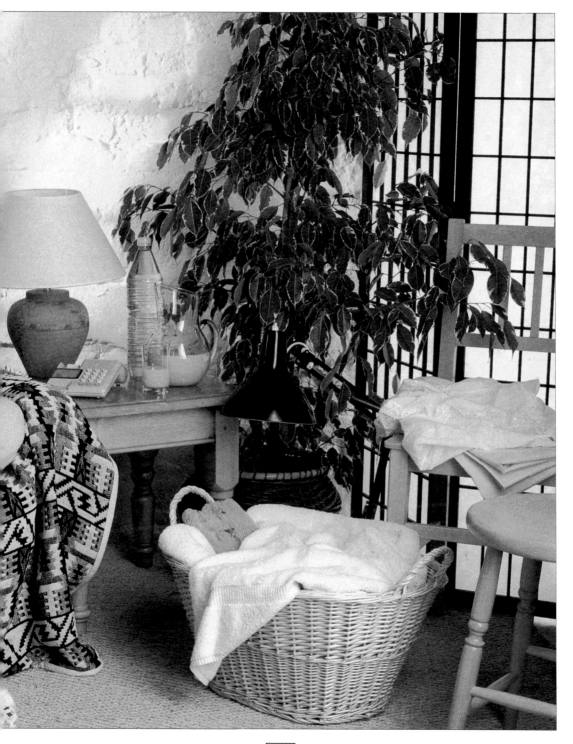

Therapies That May Help in Labor

There are a number of therapies that may help in labor. Some of these you may practice yourself, perhaps with your partner's help, others require you to have a therapist with you at the delivery. They include homeopathy, hypnotherapy, herbal treatments, aromatherapy, massage, acupressure, acupuncture and shiatsu.

Homeopathy

Labor is such an individual experience that it is not possible to talk about a best therapy for all women. Homeopathy is helpful at all stages of labor, as it deals with both the physical and mental state of the mother. You and your partner should consult your homeopath well in advance and ask them what you can do in the event of certain eventualities. You can then take your homeopathic first aid kit (see panel opposite) with you when you go into labor and your partner can administer remedies as and when required. The remedies listed here can be helpful in certain circumstances.

Hypnotherapy

Hypnotherapy is effective in alleviating pain. Ask your hypnotherapist to teach you and your partner the art of self-hypnosis and practice the technique well in advance of labor. You can then call upon it when you need it in labor.

Herbal Treatments

There are several herbal remedies that you can take throughout the first and second stages of labor. You should drink half a

Homeopathic First Aid Kit	
Treatment	Symptoms
Caulophyllum	Weakness, exhaustion and labor not proceeding
Gelsemium	Trembling and weakness
Pulsatilla	Weepy and indecisive, needing a lot of comfort. Said to help turn breech baby
Arsenicum album	Great fear and anxiety about labor*
Aconite	Sudden fright and blood loss. Also useful for the baby if it is shaking and shocked at birth, and if it retains urine*

* Seek medical attention

cupful of infusion every half-hour or so, as required, until contractions prevent any more fluid from being taken into the stomach. After that, a few sips of tea or infusion, or 5–10 drops of tincture can be placed under the tongue to bypass the stomach, every fifteen to thirty minutes.

You may have to vary the amounts and frequency of treatment depending on the speed, or lack of it, with which the labor is progressing. If things are not happening then larger doses at more frequent intervals would be recommended (for the standard dosages see Herbalism in Part One).

Acupuncture and Shiatsu

Acupuncture and shiatsu can both be very successful in the relief of fear and pain during labor. They both require the presence of an experienced practitioner who can assist you during the birth.

Hospitals are becoming increasingly aware of the advantages of this and most will now allow you to be attended by a practitioner of your choice. You must arrange this well in advance and include it in your birth plan (*see pages 122–123*).

Water Births

Water is known to have a soothing, relaxing effect on laboring women and encourages the birth canal to open. Against this background, it is becoming increasingly acceptable for women to give birth to their babies in water, and some birth centers and a few hospitals now have special birth pools. A birth pool is a deep tank lined with plastic and filled with warm water. It usually has a padded edge to lean against. Some pools are also thermostatically controlled so that the temperature of the water remains constant, eliminating the need to keep adding warm water.

The idea is that you float in warm water throughout your labor. A number of women want to come out of the water when they are pushing the baby out and giving birth. A few, however, like to stay in the water and to give birth there. Do anything that feels right for you at the time.

The First Stage of Labor

During the first stage of labor the cervix dilates, or opens, in order to allow the baby's head to pass through it. Before the normally tough and thick cervix can dilate, it must first become thin and soft. This process, known as effacement, occurs as the cervix is gradually pulled up by uterine contractions. Once the cervix has stretched, it begins to dilate with each contraction. The midwife assesses progress by saying by how many centimetres the cervix is dilated. Dilatation is usually given in increments of one centimetre. At 5cm (2in), the cervix is described as half-dilated and this means that labor is now well under way. At 10cm (4in), the cervix is fully dilated, the entire cervical canal is eliminated and the baby is already at the top of the vagina. Once that stage is reached (the beginning of the second stage of labor), the baby's arrival is imminent.

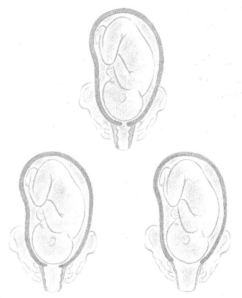

Above. *The mucus plug which stays in place throughout pregnancy has now come away, allowing the cervix to dilate gradually in response to the contractions and to the pressure exerted by the baby's head.*

Good Positions During the First Stage of Labor

During the first stage of labor, you should feel free to do whatever feels instinctively right for you. You may find yourself rocking or swaying during contractions. You may like to take a warm bath which is soothing and relaxing. A number of women like to continue moving around during this first stage of labor and then to get into their favorite position each time another contraction starts.

Take one contraction at a time and breathe your way through the contraction. Visualize your baby inside your body and what is happening to it as it moves down the birth canal. Any of the positions shown here may be right for you during this stage.

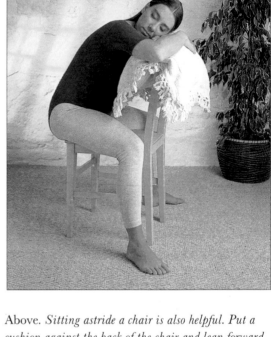

Below. *Squatting tends to assist contractions. It allows the pelvis to open as widely as possible and therefore encouraging the baby's descent. It also helps relieve any tension or pressure.*

Above. *Sitting astride a chair is also helpful. Put a cushion against the back of the chair and lean forward against it. Your body is vertical yet completely supported while your pelvis is open.*

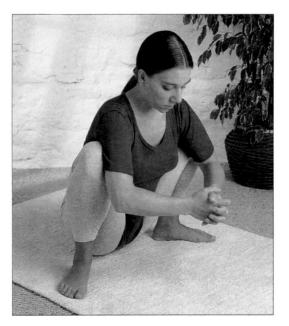

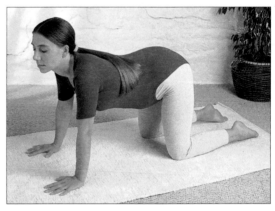

Above. *Kneel on all fours and rock backward and forward during contractions. If they become very intense, kneel forward with your head down against the floor and your bottom upward. Moving your hips around in this position may also help.*

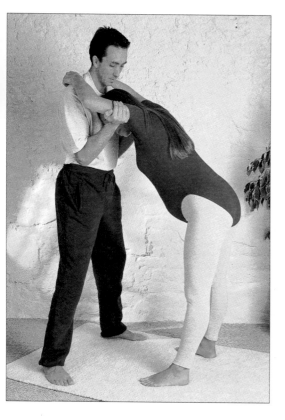

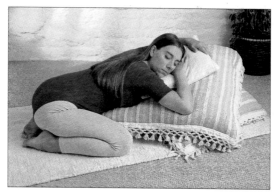

Above. *Supported kneeling is another useful position. Kneel down and support yourself by leaning forward against a nearby piece of furniture or over a pile of cushions or a big bean bag.*

Left. *Stand upright and lean slightly forward against your partner. The downward force of gravity stimulates contractions and encourages the baby's descent. You may find it helpful to circle your hips. Your partner can massage your lower back in this position, or rock you gently against him.*

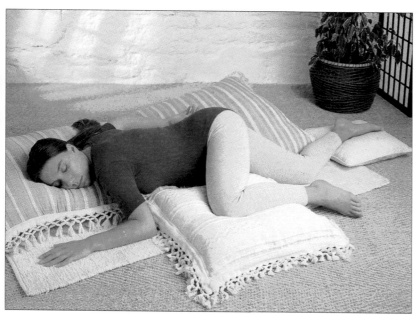

Left. *You may feel like lying down, particularly if you are getting tired. You may be most comfortable lying on your side, with your stomach well propped up by cushions. It is not a good idea to lie on your back for any length of time, except for the purposes of being examined.*

Herbal Treatments During Labor

Problem	Remedy	Effect	How Taken
Weak irregular contractions	Black cohosh Blue cohosh Raspberry leaves Southernwood Wormwood Mugwort	Tones uterus and helps establish a normal labor with strong and regular contractions	*Internally* Infusion or decoction single herb or combination; half-cup every half-hour or so Tincture; 5–10 drops under tongue every 15–30 minutes
Weak contractions, with rigid cervix	Feverfew	Equalizes circulation, makes contractions firmer and helps relieve tension in cervix	*Internally* Infusion or tincture; same dosages as above
Weak contractions	Raspberry leaves	Tones uterus, aids contractions and strengthens nerves	*Internally* Infusion; same dosage as above
Protracted labor, with waning strength of uterine muscles	Mugwort Pennyroyal Goldenseal	Strengthens contractions	*Internally* Infusion or tincture; same dosages as above
Fear, tension and pain associated with over-strong contractions	Skullcap Blue cohosh Lady's slipper Wild yam Cramp bark Black horehound Motherwort Squaw vine Yellow jasmine Raspberry leaves Black cohosh	Relaxes the uterine muscles when they are over-contracted and are thereby holding up progress of the birth. They make contractions less painful yet more productive	*Internally* Infusion/decoction or tincture; same dosages as above
Fear of pain	Essential oils of Chamomile Lavender	Relaxing, restorative to nerves	*Externally* Singly or in combination, diluted in carrier oil; 5 drops essential oil to 2 tbsp carrier oil; massage back, also feet
Pain	Essential oils of Clary sage Rose Ylang ylang Lavender Geranium Chamomile Frankincense	Relieves pain	*Externally* Massage lower back; dosages as above

The Transitional Stage

Transition comes between the end of the first stage and the beginning of the second stage of labor. It is the shortest part of labor but it can be very intense and contractions can be more painful and seem to be absolutely relentless. You may feel discouraged and worry that you cannot go on for much longer without pain relief. You may feel very emotional because you are so tired. Your legs may shake and you may shiver; you may feel irritable and bad-tempered. You may even feel nauseous. You may also get an urge to push, or bear down, though you should not do this until the midwife has examined you and has confirmed that your cervix is fully dilated. Panting a little may help you resist the urge. If you feel you just cannot go on, remember that your baby will be born soon.

Positions During Transition

It is difficult to find a comfortable position when you are in transition. Any position that you found helpful in the first stage is worth trying.

If the cervix has not yet fully dilated and you feel the urge to bear down, kneel on all fours, put your head down against the floor and your bottom up in the air. Gravity will slow the baby down in this position, while the cervix continues to dilate. This position also takes pressure off your lower back.

The Second Stage of Labor

When the cervix has opened fully, you have entered the second stage. The second stage can be over in minutes or it may take up to two hours, and ends with the birth of your long-awaited baby. You will now have an involuntary urge to push at the height of your contractions. This is a reflex, caused by the baby's head pressing on the pelvic floor and the rectum. Even if you had read nothing about giving birth, you would know instinctively when to take a deep breath, thus lowering your diaphragm and exerting pressure on the uterus, which helps to push the baby out.

Pushing is painless but hard work. It should be a smooth, continuous effort; gradual and slow so that the vaginal muscles and tissues have the chance to stretch to allow the baby's head through without tearing you or necessitating an episiotomy.

The first sign that the baby is entering the world is the bulging of the perineum and the anus. More and more of the baby's head then appears at the vaginal opening; this is called crowning. Sometimes the baby will be born very quickly at this stage, with head and body coming out in one contraction. Sometimes though, the birth may happen more slowly over a number of contractions. This depends on your position and that of the baby's head, as well as its size. If it is slow and you are in a lot of pain, the midwife will help you breathe your baby out gently in order to avoid a tear. If she feels you are likely to tear badly, she will perform an episiotomy (*see page 142*) unless you have expressed a firm desire not to have one in your birth plan. However, it is usually advisable to be guided by those caring for you at this point.

Positions for Giving Birth

Pushing is harder work if you are lying on your back because you are pushing the baby uphill in this position. An upright, or semi-upright position is therefore best for delivery, as gravity will help your efforts. Your pelvis should be open, and your pelvic floor and vaginal opening should be relaxed.

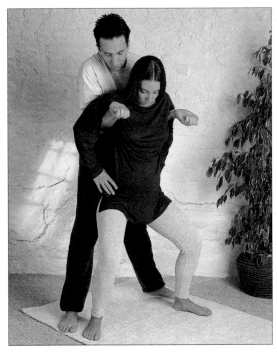

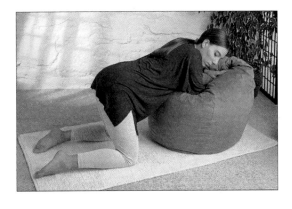

Above. *Many women give birth in a kneeling position. It eases pressure on the perineum, allowing the soft tissues to expand and stretch as the baby is born.*

Above. *Your partner stands behind you taking your weight on his arms. With each contraction, bend your knees and spread your feet apart to open the pelvis.*

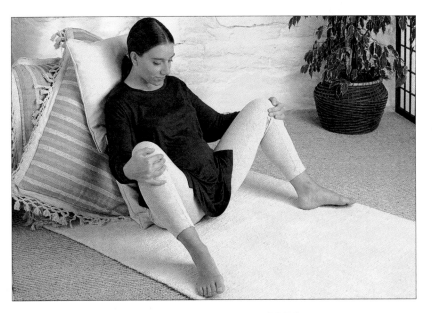

Left. *This is a common delivery position. Sit propped up against cushions, with your knees bent and apart, and your head dropped forward toward your chest. You can lean back between your contractions and rest. You will be able to see the baby being born.*

Pain Relief

Method	Stage of Labor	How Given	Does it Work?	Side-effects
Narcotics	1	Injection into vein in arm or muscle in buttocks	Timing is crucial—if given too early, effects may wear off; if too late, can prevent urge to push and can affect baby	Forceps delivery may be necessary if you cannot push. May feel drowsy or sick. Baby may be drowsy and slow to breathe, have sucking difficulties and poor muscle tone
Epidural	1, if cesarean delivery	Injected into epidural space between spinal cord and backbone of lumbar region	Usually	Chances of forceps and episiotomy are higher. Necessitates continuous fetal monitoring. May feel numbness in legs for some time after delivery. May require catheter through loss of sensation in bladder, which can lead to urinary tract infections. May cause headache
Pudendal nerve block	2, if forceps delivery is indicated	Injection through wall of vagina	Not always	None
Transcutaneous Electrical Nerve Stimulation (TENS)	1, 2	Electrodes attached to back, low-frequency current directed by the mother	Not always	None
Acupuncture	1, 2	Needles inserted into acupuncture points	Good rate of success	None
Hypnosis	1, 2	Use of self-hypnosis	Usually	None
Herbal treatment	1, 2	Massage, Raspberry leaf infusions	May not work	None
Homeopathy	1, 2	Caulophyllum orally	Usually	None
Massage	1, 2	Administered by massage therapist or partner	May relieve back pain	None
General anesthetic	If cesarean delivery	Injection	Yes	Recovery is often slow

Helping the Baby Out

In very difficult or long labor which can result in either an over-stressed baby or an exhausted mother, there are various ways of helping the baby out.

Episiotomy

An episiotomy is a cut in the perineum. A local anesthetic is given first, and a cut is made, using scissors, into the skin and muscle at the lower end of the vagina. Once the baby is out the cut is then stitched. On the whole, mothers report more drawbacks to episiotomy than advantages. Getting into a good delivery position will help mimimize the chances of episiotomy. If you would like to avoid having one, you should discuss this well in advance with the medical staff who are taking care of you and perhaps include it in your birth plan (*see page 122–123*).

Forceps

These are rather like big salad servers and are sometimes used to help the baby out in the second stage of labor, when the cervix is fully dilated and the baby's head has come down into the mother's pelvis but is not descending any further. They may also be used in cases of fetal or maternal distress.

Your legs will be put in stirrups and a local anesthetic injected into the perineum. Forceps are inserted into the vagina and the blades cupped round the sides of the baby's head, then an episiotomy is done. The idea is that you push, while the doctor pulls. Once the head is delivered, the forceps are removed and you can push the baby out normally.

Vacuum Extraction (Ventouse)

This procedure works like a miniature vacuum cleaner. A suction cup attached to a vacuum apparatus is placed on the baby's head and the baby is sucked out with each contraction as you push. The advantages of this method over forceps delivery are that the cervix does not need to be fully dilated and the mother still has to do a fair amount of the pushing. As a result it is viewed as less interventionist than forceps. The baby may have a small bump on its head rather like a large bruised blister, which subsides after a day or two.

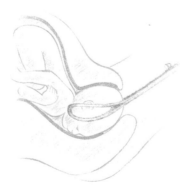

Above. *In a forceps delivery, the baby is gently helped down the vagina.*

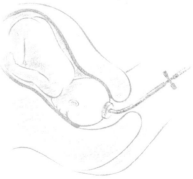

Above. *In vacuum extraction, suction aids the baby's arrival into the world.*

Cesarean

A cesarean section may be planned, or it may be an emergency procedure to halt a prolonged labor that involves risk either to mother or baby. There are various reasons for performing cesareans, including the baby's head being too big for the pelvis, some multiple births, and when the mother suffers from diseases such as hypertension, diabetes, renal disease and eclampsia. Because it involves major abdominal surgery, cesareans are not undertaken lightly. Recovery is obviously slower.

A cesarean section can be done under general anesthetic or under an epidural anesthetic, which means that you are conscious throughout and see your baby at the moment of birth.

The Third Stage of Labor

After the baby is born, the uterus rests for a short time. About fifteen minutes later, it starts to contract again, relatively painlessly, to expel the placenta and its membranes. You can help expel the placenta yourself, both by squatting and by putting the baby to the breast, which helps the uterus to contract.

The placental delivery is almost always the easiest part of giving birth, but if the placenta does not separate from the uterus, it may have to be extracted by hand. However, some women may not want this, and there are several herbal remedies that may help to bring away the placenta during this final stage of labor. They work by stimulating contractions of the uterus and so help delivery of the placenta. They may be taken in infusions, decoctions or tinctures; or simply crushed in your hands to release the volatile oils. For infusions and decoctions take half to one cupful every half-hour or so after the birth. For tinctures take 5–10 drops at the same rate until the placenta has been delivered. The most useful herbs during this stage include southernwood, wormwood, mugwort, cloves, goldenseal, rue, nutmeg, hyssop, beth root and pennyroyal.

Once the third stage of labor is accomplished, you will probably want to do nothing at all but doze, rest and gaze at the wonder of your newborn baby together with your partner.

CHAPTER SIX

After the Birth

❧

As soon as your baby is born you reach out to take this long-awaited miracle into your arms. This is a wonderful moment, and one that you will cherish for the rest of your life. However tiring your labor, it will all pale into insignificance compared to the joy and elation you will feel holding your own baby. Within just a few minutes of birth, your new baby will be able to make eye contact with you, exploring your face intently. Welcome your baby into the world with your gentle touch; skin-to-skin is the most reassuring sensation you can offer your baby. If you are planning to breastfeed, put your baby to your breast as soon as possible; instinctively your baby will latch on, already knowing how to suck. Let your baby understand right from the start that you represent safety, warmth, comfort and closeness. In this way, start as you mean to go on, providing an excellent basis on which to build a good lifelong relationship.

Getting to Know Your Baby

If you are at home for the birth, you will have plenty of time to get to know your newborn baby. If you are in hospital, with any luck you may be left alone with your partner and your baby for a while. Hospital practice varies in the way the time immediately after the birth is dealt with, and you can discuss the options with the hospital staff at your prenatal clinic. You can also state your preferences in your birth plan (*see pages 122–123*).To some extent, though, what the hospital decides to do will depend on how you and the baby are immediately after the birth.

At some point, your pulse and blood pressure will be checked and your temperature will be taken. If you have had a straightforward delivery you will probably want to go to the lavatory and you may also want a bath and a cup of tea. Some women are so exhausted and yet so at peace with themselves and their baby that all they want to do is sleep.

Is Your Baby in Good Health?

Your baby will be weighed, measured and foot-printed, then given a name band shortly after delivery. The baby's general state will also be assessed according to the Apgar score almost immediately after the birth. This involves checking five specific factors—breathing or respiratory rate, pulse rate, color (pallor), muscle tone and reflexes or response to stimuli—and points are awarded from 0 to 2 for each of the five factors. The baby who scores 10 is in good general health. Testing according to the Apgar scale may be repeated after five minutes if it is thought necessary.

What Your Baby Looks Like

Newborn babies do not usually look absolutely beautiful—except perhaps to their parents—until a few days after the birth. Do not be surprised if your baby has little bruises, puffy eyes and an elongated head, all of which are caused by pressure in the birth canal. Bruising and puffiness will disappear in a few days, and the head will regain its round shape in a couple of weeks.

Your baby may also have enlarged breasts and swollen genitals. This is perfectly normal in both girls and boys, and is caused by hormonal fluctuations which will settle down soon after the birth. The umbilical cord will be clamped and cut when it has stopped pulsating and the clamped stump at the baby's navel will be left to drop off of its own accord, usually within ten days. Before you leave hospital, the baby will be given the Guthrie test for phenylketonuria. This entails taking a small blood sample from the baby and analyzing it for a vitamin K deficiency. Phenylketonuria is a disease which, if untreated, causes a child to be mentally handicapped. If the baby is found to have the disease, it can be treated with complete success.

The Baby's First Impressions

Your baby's eyes will open soon after birth. Until a few decades ago, it was thought that babies were only sensitive to light and dark. We now know that a baby can focus on objects at a distance of around 30cm (12in), which is the perfect distance to see your features clearly when you hold the baby in your arms. At this age, the baby's most common interaction with you will be intense gazing. You will soon see that your new baby is able to express emotion by crying and frowning. Crying is a baby's most important means of communication, and you will soon learn to distinguish between your baby's cries of hunger, discomfort, pain and loneliness. Some babies seem to smile, though many people will tell you that this only indicates gas. Your baby has an enormous capacity for learning. Every cuddle, every smile, every kiss and every softly spoken word teaches your baby awareness, trust, love and pleasure. All this comes from you and your partner. Most of a baby's early learning comes through these first feeds, when touch and sensation occur simultaneously and give the baby the first impression of the world.

Bonding

You may look at your baby and instantly feel a strong bond, somewhat like love at first sight. Or you may be surprised when the baby you see is not quite the baby you had imagined or expected. Some mothers feel guilty if they do not experience instant bonding. But just because it is not love at first sight does not necessarily mean that all is lost—far from it. Your relationship with your baby is a little like an adult love affair. And, as we are all aware, love does not always happen instantly—it may simply need a little nurturing and time to grow. Each of you needs time to get used to the other, to learn to love the smell of each other and to watch for actions and reactions in the other. All of it is part of the process.

Physical Complaints

You have just gone through a physically taxing and traumatic event, and you may well be feeling sore and tired. In particular, your perineum may feel like it has just gone through a liquidizer. Although you may be offered painkillers in hospital, there are some complementary remedies which may be helpful.

Homeopathic Remedies

To help heal bruising, take *Arnica*, and to help deal with soreness, particularly if you have had a tear or an episiotomy, take *Calendula*. There are a number of remedies for exhaustion but the remedy may vary depending on the type of exhaustion. For example, exhaustion caused by hormonal changes may be rectified with *Sepia*, whereas exhaustion caused by loss of body fluids (through blood-loss and breastfeeding) may

require *China*. Because it is not an easy diagnosis to make it would be best to consult your homeopathic practitioner for further advice *(see pages 29–31)*.

Herbal Remedies

There are also several herbal remedies that will help you recuperate from the arduous experience of childbirth. The main problems you could experience immediately following delivery and the appropriate remedies are listed in the table opposite. For instructions on preparing remedies, see *Herbalism* in Part One *(pages 23–24)*.

Naturopathy

For perineal pain or after an episiotomy, alternately bathe the perineum in hot and cold water. Sea salt baths and Dead Sea mud baths are also recommended.

Herbal Remedies After Delivery

Problem	Remedy	Method of Application
Exhaustion	Lavender	**Externally** Tincture; several drops rubbed into wrists and temples and applied to nostrils
	Chinese angelica False unicorn root	**Internally** Infusion or decoction from single herb; a cupful three times daily Tincture; 5–10 drops in cup of water, three times daily
Damaged perineum	Calendula	**Externally** Tincture; a few drops added to water in bidet
	St John's wort	**Externally** Infusion added to bathwater or water in bidet **Internally** Strong infusion; one cupful twice daily
	Comfrey	**Externally** Apply poultice to scar **Internally** Infusion; one cupful three times daily
To help uterus contract	Raspberry leaves Pennyroyal Black haw Squaw vine Black cohosh	**Internally** Infusion or decoction from single herb or combination; one cupful three times daily Tincture; 5–10 drops in a cup of water, three times daily

Breast or Bottle?

You will no doubt have given plenty of thought to the breast versus bottle question well before your baby is born and will almost certainly have reached your own decision. Ultimately, it is a very personal decision, though the arguments for and against each should be considered. Decades ago, bottle-feeding was considered a convenient way of feeding your baby. It is now known, however, that breastfeeding supplies the baby with special nutrients and helps to develop its immune system. It seems to provide some protection against serious infections, especially diarrhea and other gut problems. It is also implicated in protecting babies against crib death. breastfeeding is also more convenient; there is no mixing, sterilizing and messing around with measuring, checking temperatures and reheating. At no time is this worse than in the middle of the night.

There are other advantages too; it encourages strong bonding between the mother and baby through skin-to-skin contact, the baby is less likely to get fat and it also helps the mother regain her figure by causing the release of oxytocin which helps the uterus return to its pre-pregnancy size. On the other hand, bottle-fed babies can be fed by someone else, particularly the father, which can do much to encourage bonding between them at this early stage.

Problems with Breastfeeding

Doctors now recognize that breast is best and encourage mothers to breastfeed if they can. However, help and advice about how to do it are not always so easily available. Do ask straight away if you have problems with breastfeeding. If you decide to put off asking for help when you need it, you may be faced with a vicious circle; you find breastfeeding difficult and painful, your baby is frustrated and hungry from not receiving enough milk and this makes you feel guilty and worried, which in turn makes you tense and unable to relax properly while you are trying to feed your baby.

Technique is all important and it does not always come naturally. Many women have had problems with feeding their babies—so do not hesitate to ask for advice at the hospital, or from your midwife, health visitor or GP. They should also be able to refer you to a breastfeeding counselor or specialist self-help group within your area which offers support and help (*see page 157 for organizations*).

Insufficient Milk Sometimes the milk supply seems to be inadequate for the baby's needs and the mother begins to worry about it, which in turn leads to less milk production—a vicious circle that is difficult to break. Tension, exhaustion and general stress do not help with adequate milk pro-

duction. In addition, the baby may not be sucking hard enough from the start—milk is produced and "let down" by the trigger of of this sucking. Or the mother may not be feeding the baby often enough, in which case the undrunk milk distends the milk glands, preventing further milk production. This is why demand feeding is best for both mother and baby. The more your baby drinks, the more milk you will produce.

While you are breastfeeding you should eat good, nutritious food and drink plenty of fluids. Herbal teas such as borage, holy thistle, nettles, vervain, raspberry leaves, comfrey, marshmallow, fennel or dill will help stimulate the production of milk.

Sore and Cracked Nipples To avoid this very common problem, it is best to prepare the nipples before the baby is born. During the last few months of your pregnancy, rub the breasts and nipples firmly with a rough towel, rolling the nipples between the fingers to toughen the skin. Then apply calendula cream or a chamomile-based ointment.

The nipples may become cracked and sore because the baby is sucking the nipple rather than taking the whole areola into the mouth. Make sure that the baby latches on properly. If your nipples are very sore it may help if you express milk manually for a few days until they heal.

Engorgement This happens if the breasts become over-full; it is usually caused by the baby not feeding frequently enough, or feeding too long from one breast. A baby can empty a breast in under seven minutes, and one breast should never be sucked for longer than twelve minutes. Feed the baby equally from both breasts at each feed.

Blocked Milk Duct Sometimes the outlet to one of the milk ducts becomes blocked. This can be the result of a tight or badly fitting bra pressing on a milk gland, or by your milk becoming unusually thick, which can prevent a duct from emptying fully. If you have a blocked duct, you will probably have a lump in the breast; this may become infected, painful and make you feverish.

If you develop a blocked duct feed your baby frequently, as the sucking will help clear it. Move the baby regularly so that every part of the nipple gets stimulated. Try heating the breast gently with a warm compress before you feed the baby which may loosen any dried milk that is blocking the outlet of the duct. You might also try expressing and massaging in a hot bath to clear the blockage. Get plenty of rest, eat well and drink lots of fluids to increase milk production.

It may also help to massage the breast after each feeding. The ducts that carry the milk run from the outside of the breasts toward the nipples, rather like the spokes of a wheel. Holding the fingers close together, massage in a downward motion, from the outside toward the nipples.

Mastitis This occurs when infection enters the breast, usually through a cracked nipple. The breast becomes engorged, hard, red, tender and painful. If the condition is caught early enough, it is usually possible to avoid it becoming any worse by having the baby feed more often from the affected breast. It is important to continue using that breast. It is equally important to seek medical help if mastitis continues.

Breast Abscess If mastitis is not properly treated, it can develop into a painful, pus-filled abscess, which may cause a fever. Again, it is very important that you seek medical attention. One method of treatment is to take a course of antibiotics in the early stages, although this may cause diarrhea in the baby. If it does not respond to treatment, you may need to have it drained surgically under general anesthetic.

Therapies for Breast Problems

There are a number of therapies that may be of great help in easing some of the more common breast problems associated with breastfeeding.

Herbal Treatments

To prevent sore nipples from occurring, apply buttermilk and honey, or comfrey ointment, to keep the nipple supple. Alternatively, you can use calendula or chickweed ointment, thin honey, almond oil or rosewater.

For breast engorgement, essential oils of fennel and lavender are particularly useful. Add a few drops of oil to a bowl of hot water, disperse well and then wring a wash cloth out in the water and apply frequently to the breast. Wash the breast thoroughly before feeding to remove traces of oil which may be too stimulating or powerful for a very small baby.

You can also try placing a well-washed, fresh rhubarb or cabbage leaf inside your bra for about three hours. After this time, the breast will have returned to its normal size and you will be able to nurse properly once more.

Acute mastitis can be treated with poultices of a mixture of chopped comfrey leaves and some crushed flaxseed: pound into a paste with hot water, then put in a muslin bag and apply to the affected area.

Homeopathic Remedies for Breast Problems

Problem	In Detail	Remedy
Insufficient milk flow	Milk flow is unsatisfactory because the mother is emotionally distressed	*Ignatia*
Slow milk flow	The breasts are getting smaller and the mother is depressed and despondent, and feels thirsty all the time	*Lac defloratum*
Cracked nipples	Sore cracked nipples	*Castor equus*
Engorged breasts	Hot, throbbing, red-streaked breasts	*Belladonna*
Engorged breasts	Hard breasts, worse when any pressure is applied, and on movement *	*Bryonia*
Engorged breasts	Hard, sensitive breasts. Abscesses. Pains in the nipples radiating all over the body when the baby feeds *	*Phytollaca*
Mastitis	Painful lump in breast and start of mastitis *	*Bryonia 30*—take every 2 hours and see your practitioner if no improvement after three doses.

* Seek medical attention

Infusions, decoctions or tinctures of dandelion root, cleavers, echinacea or calendula and garlic capsules taken internally are also useful. For local relief, apply distilled witch hazel to the area, or bathe with an infusion of marshmallow flowers and leaves.

Massage

If engorgement develops, the affected breast can be gently massaged in a bath of warm soapy water. The warmth of the water will encourage the milk to flow out into the bath, relieving some of the pressure on the breasts. As mentioned earlier, massage the breasts from the chest toward the nipples, thus encouraging the milk down the ducts.

Diet While Breastfeeding

Unless a woman is very badly nourished, or has been ill or suffered pregnancy complications, she will probably produce enough good-quality milk. Breastfeeding uses 300–500 calories a day, much of which is supplied by the fat reserves built up during pregnancy. When you are breastfeeding, you must eat a nutritious, balanced diet and be sure to drink plenty of liquids. You may well experience great thirst while the baby is feeding, so perhaps make yourself a drink to have while you are feeding.

Reread the section on *Diet* in Part One to refresh your memory and continue to eat a sensible diet. You will need to consume about 500 extra calories a day to sustain breastfeeding. Many women find that they are hungrier when they are breastfeeding and it should be enough to allow yourself to be guided by your hunger without following any special diet.

You will also need plenty of extra fluid, and here your thirst is your best guide. Drink mineral water, herbal teas and fresh fruit juices diluted with water.

Eat unrefined, unprocessed foods rich in vitamins and minerals. Make sure that you are taking in enough calcium to replace the calcium you lose in your breast milk, and make sure that your intake of iron is adequate by eating plenty of iron-rich foods.

Some of everything that you eat, drink or absorb in any other way finds its way into your bloodstream and then into your milk. It is therefore advisable to avoid anything that might harm your baby, or to which your baby might react with indigestion or gas. If you are taking any form of medication, check with your doctor that it will not affect your baby. Avoid cigarettes, alcohol, coffee, chocolate, citrus fruits and strawberries, all of which may affect the baby.

Going Home

You will probably be delighted to relax in your normal environment once again, but it is possible, at the same time, that the newness and the responsibility of your changed circumstances combine to make you feel a little overwhelmed. This is particularly common with a first baby. It is caused partly by the action of your hormones as they settle down again to their normal levels, and partly because everything is so new.

The baby only seems to have two preoccupations at this time—breast and bowel—and you may feel that this constant demand for feeding and diaper changes is just too much. This stage does not usually last for more than about six weeks, but even that can seem like a very long time. If anything is worrying you at all, it is particularly important that you talk to your health care practitioner.

Meanwhile, do not concentrate so much on your baby that you neglect yourself or your partner. Think about your own diet and your need for rest, and save a little time in your busy schedule for yourself and your partner who, understandably, may feel a little overshadowed by the arrival of the newest member of your family.

Postnatal Depression

Most women feel nothing but elation and satisfaction at the birth of their babies, but some new mothers feel depressed and helpless. Postnatal depression—known in its mildest form as postpartum blues—is common after the birth of a baby.

You may feel especially sensitive and weep easily. You may also experience mood swings, which are hard either to understand or to cope with. If you do feel awful, it is important that you confide in someone. Do not be ashamed of your feelings or think you are a failure. Talk to your doctor, your health visitor or your partner—whoever you feel is most approachable.

There are various therapies that can help with postnatal depression. Taking B vitamins in the form of brewer's yeast will help your nervous system. Drink teas of rosemary, vervain, wild oats, borage, St John's wort and celery seed, and use essential oils of clary sage and ylang ylang, either as massage oils, on your pillow or in the bath. Homeopathy is also successful with postnatal depression, though it can be such a difficult condition to treat that it is generally better to consult a homeopath than to try self-treatment.

Herbal Baths for the Baby

Your baby will greatly benefit from herb-scented baths which can be both soothing and restorative at a time when the baby is having to adapt to the outside world and all the new sensations that entails. Make up an infusion to add to the baby's bathwater of one or a combination of the following herbs: rose petals, lavender flowers, geranium, meadowsweet, rosemary or jasmine (*see Herbal Baths on page 24*).

Baby Massage

Babies enjoy being massaged regularly from a very early age. Some parents worry that they might injure their baby if they massage them, but this is highly unlikely, and in any case, the baby will soon let you know if you cause any discomfort. Choose a warm room, with low lighting. Peaceful music can enhance a calm and loving atmosphere too.

A light dusting of cornstarch or a thin layer of pure vegetable oil such as almond or olive oil will make your hands glide over the baby's skin more easily and will be more comfortable for the baby.

You can massage virtually any part of your baby's body, using very gentle pressure of the fingertips and occasionally squeezing the muscles with your whole hand. A small baby's attention span is relatively short, so any massage sequence should consist of only a few repetitions before you change to a new movement.

You and your partner can now enjoy your new baby, getting to know this small person who will change your lives in the most unexpected and delightful ways. This is the beginning of the most profound relationship you may ever experience, and different in many ways from the relationship and love you share with your partner.

Common Complaints and Therapies for the Three Trimesters of Pregnancy

Complaint	Cause	Symptoms	Therapy
Abdominal pain **Trimester:** 3	Ligaments supporting uterus stretch because of pregnancy hormones	Cramp-like pains in abdomen or dragging pain down one side	Aromatherapy, color therapy, homeopathy, massage, osteopathy, hot-water bottle to relax muscles
Backache **Trimesters:** 1, 2, 3	Hormones of pregnancy cause a general softening of the ligaments, particularly in the pelvic area. The fetus presses on nerves in the pelvis	Ache across the lower back	Alexander technique, aromatherapy, color therapy, chiropractic, herbal treatment, homeopathy, massage, osteopathy, shiatsu, yoga
Bleeding gums **Trimesters:** 1, 2, 3	Increased blood supply to all parts of the body, together with increasingly soft gums because of pregnancy hormones	Gums bleed easily on brushing teeth or eating particularly hard foods	Herbal treatment, homeopathy, naturopathy
Breathlessness **Trimesters:** 3	Baby pushes against the diaphragm	Shortness of breath, especially on exertion	Acupressure, acupuncture, Alexander technique, naturopathy, yoga
Constipation **Trimesters:** 1, 2, 3	Hormones of pregnancy may slow down bowel movements. Insufficient fiber in diet, and not drinking enough liquids	Irregular bowel movements, with small hard stools	Acupressure, acupuncture, aromatherapy, color therapy, chiropractic, herbal treatment, homeopathy, massage, naturopathy, osteopathy, reflexology, shiatsu, yoga
Cramps **Trimesters:** 3	Probably caused by low levels of calcium in blood-stream	Sudden pains in legs and feet. Can sometimes be bad enough at night to wake you up	Aromatherapy, color therapy, herbal treatment, homeopathy, massage, naturopathy, shiatsu, yoga

Bold numbers under each complaint refer to the trimesters in which it might occur.

Common Complaints and Therapies for the Three Trimesters of Pregnancy (cont)

Complaint	Cause	Symptoms	Therapy
Cystitis **Trimesters:** **1, 2, 3**	Softening of bladder wall predisposes it to infection	Frequent desire to urinate, with discomfort and pain	Acupressure, acupuncture, color therapy, herbal treatment, homeopathy, naturopathy, shiatsu
Dizziness **Trimester:** **3**	Demands of uterus for increased blood supply may cause brain to be relatively and temporarily deprived of blood. Anemia can also cause dizziness	Head may spin, particularly on getting up too quickly. May need to sit or lie down	Acupressure, acupuncture, Alexander technique, color therapy, herbal treatment, homeopathy, massage, naturopathy, shiatsu, yoga
Edema **Trimster:** **3**	Fluid retention in body. Pressure of uterus on blood vessels returning blood to heart	Swelling in hands and ankles. Shoes and rings may feel tight, fingers stiff in morning	Acupressure, acupuncture, aromatherapy, color therapy, herbal treatment, homeopathy, massage, naturopathy, shiatsu
Fatigue **Trimesters:** **1, 2, 3**	Common symptom of pregnancy due to anxiety, lack of sleep, weight of baby (see insomnia)	Need for more sleep than usual, inability to do as much as before, falling asleep at odd times. Legs sometimes ache and unwilling to carry you any further	Acupressure, acupuncture, Alexander technique, aromatherapy, color therapy, herbal treatment, homeopathy, massage, meditation, naturopathy, reflexology, shiatsu, yoga
Flatulence **Trimesters:** **1, 2, 3**	The intestine is more sluggish than usual and gas may be more difficult to expel	Distended stomach, rumbling tummy and frequent passing of gas	Color therapy, herbal treatment, homeopathy, massage, naturopathy, reflexology
Frequent urination **Trimesters:** **1, 2, 3**	Increased blood supply causes bladder to become irritable and to empty itself more often	Urgent need to pass urine at frequent intervals in day and night	Herbal treatment, homeopathy

Bold numbers under each complaint refer to the trimesters in which it might occur.

Common Complaints and Therapies for the Three Trimesters of Pregnancy (cont)

Complaint	Cause	Symptoms	Therapy
Groin and low back pain **Trimesters: 2, 3**	Ligaments supporting uterus stretch because of pregnancy hormones, causing general softening of ligaments	Cramp-like pains in abdomen, or dragging pain down one side	Aromatherapy, massage, hot-water bottle to relax muscles
Heartburn **Trimesters: 2, 3**	Half of all pregnant women experience heartburn toward end of second trimester. It is related to effect of increased hormones of pregnancy, which soften valve in digestive tract, so that acid rises from the stomach	A sudden burning sensation in throat or at top of stomach. Frequently accompanied by regurgitation of small amounts of sour, acid fluid. Often worse at night	Homeopathy, yoga
Hemorrhoids **Trimesters: 2, 3**	Relaxing effect of pregnancy hormones on rectal veins and increased pressure in abdomen caused by baby's head in pelvis obstructing blood vessels in rectum. More common if piles run in the family	Itchiness around rectum and pain when passing stools with possible slight bleeding	Acupressure, acupuncture, aromatherapy, chiropractic, herbal treatment, massage, naturopathy, osteopathy, shiatsu, yoga
Incontinence **Trimester: 3**	Pressure of enlarging uterus on bladder results in inability of pelvic floor muscles to prevent leakage	Involuntary urination, particularly when you cough, sneeze or laugh	Acupressure, acupuncture, color therapy, herbal treatment, homeopathy, hypnotherapy, massage, meditation, naturopathy, reflexology, shiatsu, yoga
Insomnia **Trimesters: 1, 2, 3**	Increase in metabolism, frequent need to urinate may wake you up	Inability to go to sleep, waking up at night and inability to go back to sleep	Acupressure, acupuncture, herbal treatment, homeopathy, naturopathy

Bold numbers under each complaint refer to the trimesters in which it might occur.

Common Complaints and Therapies for the Three Trimesters of Pregnancy (cont)

Complaint	Cause	Symptoms	Therapy
Morning sickness **Trimesters:**	The sudden high level of hormones, particularly HCG, can bring on nausea	Nauseous feelings, particularly at slight or smell of food, sometimes accompanied by vomiting	Acupressure, acupuncture, color therapy, herbal treatment, homeopathy, shiatsu, yoga
Pelvic discomfort **Trimester:** **3**	Baby's head pressing on nerves, especially when head is engaged in pelvic cavity	Pain in groin and where pubic bones meet at the front, particularly after exercise	Acupressure, acupuncture, massage
Stretch marks **Trimesters:** **2, 3**	Poor nutrition or excess weight gain can cause collagen bundles to tear as skin stretches to accommodate your burgeoning shape	Wavy, pinkish silvery marks occur on the breasts, abdomen, thighs and buttocks	Aromatherapy, herbal treatment
Sweating **Trimesters:** **2, 3**	Increased blood supply to all parts of body, which causes blood vessels to dilate	Feeling hot and sweaty, especially on exercise and at night	Color therapy, herbal treatment, naturopathy,
Thrush **Trimesters:** **1, 2, 3**	The yeast *Candida albicans*, which affects the vagina, can be more common in pregnancy	Thick white discharge, intense itching, and sometimes pain on passing urine	Color therapy, herbal treatment, homeopathy, naturopathy, reflexology
Varicose veins **Trimesters:** **1, 2, 3**	Common in pregnancy and more likely if varicose veins run in the family	Irritated, itchy skin, together with dull ache	Alexander technique, aromatherapy, herbal treatment, homeopathy, massage, naturopathy, yoga

Bold numbers under each complaint refer to the trimesters in which it might occur.

Useful Addresses

Please enclose a stamped addressed envelope with all enquiries.

MATERNITY CARE

American College of Nurse-Midwives
818 Connecticut Avenue N.W.
Suite 900
Washington, DC 20006
Tel: (202) 728 9860
Fax: (202) 728 9897

WOMEN'S HEALTH

Boston Women's Health Book Collective
PO Box 192
Somerville, MA 02144
Tel: (617) 625 0277

National Black Women's Health Project
1237 Gordon Street, S.W.
Atlanta, GA 30310
Tel: (404) 753 0916

National Women's Health Network
514 10th Street N.W.
Suite 400
Washington, DC 20004
Tel: (202) 347 1140
Fax: (202) 347 1168

COMPLEMENTARY THERAPIES

American Holistic Medical Association
4101 Lake Boone Trail
Suite 201
Raleigh, NC 27607
Tel: (919) 787 5181
Fax: (919) 787 4916

American Holistic Nurses Association
4101 Lake Boone Trail
Suite 201
Raleigh, NC 27607
Tel: 1 800 278 AHNA

American Preventive Medical Association
459 Walker Road
Great Falls, VA 22066
Tel: (800) 230 2762
Fax: (703) 759 6711

Acupuncture

American Association of Acupuncture and Oriental Medicine
4101 Lake Boone Trail
Suite 201
Raleigh, NC 27607
Tel: (919) 787 5181

National Commission for the Certification of Acupuncturists
1424 16th Street, N.W. #501
Washington, DC 20036
Tel: (202) 232 1404

Acupressure

Acupressure Institute
1533 Shattuck Avenue
Berkeley, CA 94709
Tel: (510) 845 1059
Fax: (510) 845 1496

Alexander Technique

North American Society of Teachers of the Alexander Technique
PO Box 5536
Playa del Rey, CA 90296
Tel: (800) 473 0620

Aromatherapy

National Association for Holistic Aromatherapists
219 Carl Street
San Francisco,
CA 94117–3804
Tel: (415) 564 6799

Chiropractic

American Chiropractic Association
1701 Clarendon Blvd.
Arlington, VA 22209
Tel: (703) 276 8800

Association for Network Chiropractic Spinal Analysis
PO Box 7682
Longmont, CO 80501
Tel: (303) 678 8086

International Chiropractors Association (ICA)
1110 N. Glebe Road, Suite 1000
Arlington, VA 22201

Tel: (800) 423 4690
Fax: (703) 528 5023

Herbalism

American Herbalists Guild
3411 Cunnison Lane
Soquel, CA 95073
Tel: (403) 438 1700

American Herb Association
PO Box 1673
Nevada City, CA 95959
Tel: (916) 265 9552

Homeopathy

Homeopathic Academy of Naturopathic Physicians
14653 South Graves Road
Mulino, OR 97042
Tel: (503) 829 7326

National Center for Homeopathy
801 N. Fairfax Street, Suite 306
Alexandria, VA 22314
Tel: (703) 548 7790

Hypnotherapy

American Association of Professional Hypnotherapists
PO Box 29
Boones Mill, VA 24065
Tel: (703) 334 3035

International Medical and Dental Hypnotherapy Association
4110 Edgeland, Suite 800
Royal Oaks, MI 48073–2251
Tel: (810) 549 5594

Massage

American Massage Therapy Association
820 Davis Street, Suite 100
Evanston, IL 60201–4444
Tel: (708) 864 0123

Associated Bodywork and Massage Professionals
28677 Buffalo Park Road
Evergreen, CO 80439–7347
Tel: (800) 458 2267

Naturopathy

American Association of Naturopathic Physicians

2366 Eastlake Avenue
Suite 322
Seattle, WA 98102
Tel: (206) 323 7610

American Naturopathic Association
1413 K Street, First Floor
Washington, DC 20005
Tel: (202) 682 7352

American Naturopathic Medical Association
PO Box 96273
Las Vegas, NV 89193
Tel: (702) 897 7053

Osteopathy

American Osteopathic Association
142 East Ontario Street
Chicago, IL 60611
Tel: (312) 280 5800
Fax: (312) 280 3860

Reflexology

International Institute of Reflexology
PO Box 12642
St. Petersburg,
FL 33733–2642
Tel: (813) 343 4811

Shiatsu

American Oriental Bodywork Association
6801 Jericho Turnpike
Syosset, NY 11791
Tel: (516) 364 5533
Fax: (516) 364 5559

Visualization

International Imagery Association
PO Box 1046
Bronx, NY 10471

Yoga

International Association of Yoga Therapists
109 Hillside Avenue
Mill Valley, CA 94941
Tel: (415) 383 4587
Fax: (415) 381 0876

Further Reading

Acupressure for Common Ailments, Chris Jarmey and John Tindall, London, Gaia Books, 1991

Acupuncture: Cure of Many Diseases, Felix Mann, Oxford, Butterworth-Heinemann, 1971

The Alexander Technique, Judith Leibowitz and Bill Connington, New York, HarperCollins, 1990

The Alexander Technique Birth Book: a Guide to Better Pregnancy, Natural Birth and Parenthood, Ilana Machover, Angela Drake & Jonathan Drake, London, Robinson Publishing, 1993

Alternative Medicine: a Guide to Natural Therapies, Dr Andrew Stanway, London, Bloomsbury Books, 1992

Aromatherapy: a Complete Guide to the Healing Art, Kathi Keville and Mindy Green, Fredom, CA, Crossing Press, 1995

Aromatherapy for Women and Children: Pregnancy and Childbirth, Jane Dye, Saffron Walden, C. W. Daniel, 1992

Birth-Tech: Tests and Technology in Pregnancy and Birth, Anne Charlish, New York, Facts on File, 1991

The Book of Massage, Lucinda Lidell, New York, Simon and Schuster, 1984

The Book of Yoga: the Complete Step-by-step Guide, The Sivananda Yoga Centre, London, Ebury Press, 1983

Breastfeeding your Baby, Sheila Kitzinger, New York, Alfred A. Knopf (a Dorling Kindersley book), 1995

Colour Therapy, Mary Anderson, San Francisco, Aquarian Press (an imprint of HarperCollins), 1979

Colour Therapy: the Use of Colour for Health and Healing, Pauline Wills, Dorset, Element Books, 1993

The Complete Book of Massage, Clare Maxwell-Hudson, London, Dorling Kindersley, 1988

The Complete Natural Health Consultant, Michael van Straten, London, Ebury Press, 1987

The Encyclopedia of Alternative Health Care, Kristin Olsen, London, Piatkus, 1989

The Encyclopedia of Pregnancy and Birth, Janet Balaskas and Yehudi Gordon, London, Little Brown, 1992

Get into Shape after Childbirth: Easy to Follow Routines to Tone, Trim and Relax, Gillian Fletcher, London, Ebury Press, 1991

Getting Pregnant: the Complete Guide to Fertility and Infertility, Professor Robert Winston, London, Pan Books, 1993

Giving Birth: Alternatives in Childbirth, Barbara Katz Rothman, New York, Penguin, 1982

The Healing Herbs, Michael Castleman, Emmaus, PA, Rodale Press, 1991

The Herbal for Mother and Child, Anne McIntyre, Dorset, Element Books, 1992

Homebirth, Sheila Kitzinger, New York, Dorling Kindersley, 1991

Homeopathy for Pregnancy, Birth, and your Baby's First Year, Miranda Castro, New York, St Martin's Press, 1993

Massage for Common Ailments, Sara Thomas, New York, Simon and Schuster, 1988

Natural Pregnancy, Janet Balaskas, New York, Interlink Books, 1990

New Active Birth: a Concise Guide to Natural Childbirth, Janet Balaskas, London, Thorsons, 1991

The New Our Bodies, Ourselves, The Boston Women's Health Book Collective, New York, Simon and Schuster, 1992

The New Pregnancy and Childbirth, Sheila Kitzinger, London, Penguin, 1989

Positive Pregnancy Fitness, Sylvia Klein Olkin, Garden City Park, New York, Avery Publishing Group, 1987

Pregnancy Day–by–day: a Unique Pregnancy Planner and Information–packed Guide, Sheila Kitzinger, London, Dorling Kindersley, 1990

Preparing for Birth with Yoga, Janet Balaskas, Dorset, Element Books, 1994

Water Birth: the Concise Guide to Using Water During Pregnancy, Janet Balaskas and Yehudi Gordon, Birth and Infancy, London, Thorsons, 1992

What to Expect when you're Expecting, Arlene Eisenberg, Heidi C. Murkoff, and Sandee E. Hathaway, New York, Workman Publishing Co., 1991

The Year after Childbirth, Sheila Kitzinger, New York, Charles Scribner's Sons, 1994

Yoga for Common Ailments, Drs R. Nagarathna, H. R. Nagenda and Robin Monro, London, Gaia Books, 1990

Yoga for Pregnancy, Sandra Jordan, New York, St Martin's Press, 1987

Index

ACKNOWLEDGEMENTS

I would like to offer my sincere and heartfelt thanks to all the consultants who have assisted me with the text: Donald Gibb, Debbie Shapiro, Isabelle Hughes, Ilana Machover, Anne McIntyre, Caroline Schuck, Michael van Straten and Pauline Wills. Lucy Allen's computer skills have been an enormous help and the fact that she was pregnant at the time of writing with her son, Louis, brought illuminating insights. I would also like to make a special acknowledge-

ment to Anne Johnson, whose support, encouragement and attention to detail have proved invaluable.

EDDISON SADD would like to thank John Lewis, Oxford Street, for the loan of props; we would also like to thank our models: Mia Hutchinson, Simona Mitterer and Emma Smith.

The photograph on page 84 is reproduced with kind permission from Bubbles/John Garrett.

EDDISON·SADD EDITIONS

Project Editor.................. Zoë Hughes
Copy-editor..................... Marilyn Inglis
Proofreader..................... Nikky Twyman
Indexer............................ Dorothy Frame

Art Editor........................ Pritty Ramjee
Mac Designer.................. Brazzle Atkins
Photographer.................. Gill Orsman
Illustrator....................... Julie Carpenter
Production....................... Hazel Kirkman, Charles James